Kostoris Library Christie

R02439W4988

3447

The effects of cancer treatment on reproductive functions

nce on management

Report of a Working Party
November 2007

THIS BOOK BELONGS TO:
Kostoris Library
Christie Hospital NHS Trust
Manchester
M20 4BX
Phone: 0161 446 3452

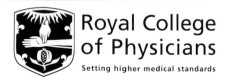 **Royal College of Physicians**
Setting higher medical standards

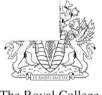 The Royal College of Radiologists

 Royal College of Obstetricians and Gynaecologists
Setting standards to improve women's health

Acknowledgements

The Working Party is grateful for the comments provided by the British Fertility Society, Cancerbackup, the Human Fertility and Embryology Authority, the Lymphoma Association, the Lymphoma Trust (Professor David Linch), Maggie's Centres, Marilyn Crawshaw, University of York, the Royal College of Paediatrics and Child Health, the Society for Endocrinology (Professor Frederick Wu), Teenage and Young Adults with Cancer Board.

The Royal College of Physicians

The Royal College of Physicians plays a leading role in the delivery of high quality patient care by setting standards of medical practice and promoting clinical excellence. We provide physicians in the United Kingdom and overseas with education, training and support throughout their careers. As an independent body representing over 20,000 Fellows and Members worldwide, we advise and work with government, the public, patients and other professions to improve health and healthcare.

Citation for this document: Royal College of Physicians, The Royal College of Radiologists, Royal College of Obstetricians and Gynaecologists. *The effects of cancer treatment on reproductive functions: Guidance on management.* Report of a Working Party. London: RCP, 2007.

Copyright

All rights reserved. No part of this publication may be reproduced in any form (including photocopying or storing it in any medium by electronic means and whether or not transiently or incidentally to some other use of this publication) without the written permission of the copyright owner. Applications for the copyright owner's written permission to reproduce any part of this publication should be addressed to the publisher.

Copyright © 2007 Royal College of Physicians

ISBN 978-1-86016-327-2

Review date: 2012

Royal College of Physicians
11 St Andrews Place, London NW1 4LE
www.rcplondon.ac.uk
Registered Charity No 210508

The Royal College of Radiologists
38 Portland Place, London W1N 4JQ
www.rcr.ac.uk

Royal College of Obstetricians and Gynaecologists
27 Sussex Place, Regent's Park, London NW1 4RG
www.rcog.org.uk

Typeset by Dan-Set Graphics, Telford, Shropshire

Printed in Great Britain by The Lavenham Press, Sudbury, Suffolk

Contents

Members of the Working Party

Graham (Ben) Mead FRCR FRCP (*Chair*)
Consultant in Medical Oncology, Southampton General Hospital, Southampton

Richard Anderson PhD FRCOG
Professor of Clinical Reproductive Science and Consultant in Reproductive Medicine,
University of Edinburgh

Chris Barratt
Professor of Reproductive Biology, University of Birmingham

Anna Cassoni FRCP FRCR
Consultant Clinical Oncologist, UCL Hospitals, London

Robert Coleman FRCP
Professor of Medical Oncology, Cancer Research Centre, Weston Park Hospital, Sheffield

Hilary Critchley FRCOG
Professor of Reproductive Medicine and Consultant Gynaecologist, University of Edinburgh

Adam Glaser FRCPCH
Consultant Paediatric and Adolescent Oncologist, Leeds Teaching Hospital

Elizabeth Hill
Lay Member, Royal College of Radiologists Patients' Liaison Group

Sol Mead
Lay Member, Royal College of Radiologists Patients' Liaison Group

John Radford FRCP
Professor of Medical Oncology, Christie Hospital, Manchester

Pawan Randev MRCGP
General Practitioner, Measham Medical Unit, Derbyshire

Simon Rule FRCP FRCPath
Consultant Haematologist, Derriford Hospital, Plymouth

Elaine Sugden FRCR
Consultant in Clinical Oncology, Churchill Hospital, Oxford

Peter Trainer FRCP
Consultant in Endocrinology, Christie Hospital, Manchester

Foreword

Although cancer predominantly affects people after they have completed their families, an important minority are diagnosed at a younger age. For example, around 11,000 patients in the age group 15–40 years are diagnosed with cancer each year in the UK. This represents around 4% of all cases of cancer. Of particular relevance in this age group are patients with breast, cervical and testicular cancers, sarcomas, leukaemias and lymphoma.

These patients have to deal not only with the impact of having cancer and the immediate consequences of treatment, but also with the possibility that surgery, radiotherapy or chemotherapy may cause gonadal damage and infertility.

The management of gonadal toxicity resulting from cancer treatment has moved on considerably in recent years. I therefore warmly welcome this report which updates a previous report published in 1998. Members of the multidisciplinary expert working party who prepared the report are to be congratulated for their clear and comprehensive summary of the state of knowledge in this area and the implications for patient care within the NHS.

I strongly commend this report to clinicians and clinical service managers involved in cancer care. The report should be equally valuable to commissioners of NHS services and to funders of future research in this field.

As survival rates following the treatment of cancer continue to improve it is essential that we should focus attention on issues related to survivorship. Fertility after treatment is clearly one such issue.

November 2007

Professor Mike Richards
National Cancer Director

Summary and recommendations

Summary

Male and female gonadal toxicity are common complications of modern anti-cancer treatments. Although effective cancer therapy, and where possible cure, are of paramount importance, infertility and hypogonadism can be a source of considerable distress. The gonadotoxic effects of radiotherapy and the older chemotherapy regimens are well described. However, a profusion of new drugs and antibodies are now in routine use with poorly validated gonadal toxic effects.

It should be noted that chemotherapy drugs are also used in some non-malignant diseases. The comments in this report also apply to this group.

All patients with reproductive potential requiring anti-cancer treatment should be fully informed prior to treatment about the possible gonadal toxic consequences of any given treatment approach, and this discussion should be documented. These discussions should take place in private, should involve appropriate family or other individuals, and whenever possible should be conducted by experienced, preferably trained, staff.

Spermatogenesis is highly sensitive to the effects of chemotherapy and irradiation and male patients should, where relevant, routinely be offered sperm banking before treatment starts. Where sperm are absent from the ejaculate, testicular sperm extraction can sometimes be successful.

Testosterone deficiency in males is a less common complication of treatment but easily correctable with testosterone replacement.

The ovary is also sensitive to cancer treatments. When there is a possibility of gonadal damage, methods of preserving fertility should be discussed.

Where there is a partner and sufficient time, embryos can often be successfully generated and stored using *in vitro* fertilisation (IVF) techniques. Egg and ovarian tissue storage are also technically feasible; however, very few successful pregnancies have been reported. The latter techniques are not currently widely available and it is recommended that a service should be developed in the context of research studies.

Uterine function can be particularly damaged by irradiation and the late effects of this treatment may affect subsequent pregnancy.

Premature menopause is a common complication of anti-cancer treatment and, depending on the context, should be treated with hormone replacement.

This document seeks to describe the patient population who are at risk and current concepts in the preemptive management and management of gonadal toxicity. We also discuss developments that are likely in the next five to ten years.

Recommendations

1   All patients with reproductive potential who require anti-cancer treatment either for cancer treatment or benign indications should be fully informed about potential gonadotoxic side effects at the time of diagnosis and prior to potentially gonadotoxic treatment. Alternative treatment strategies causing less gonadal damage should be discussed where relevant.

2   Discussion and advice given about gonadal toxicity should be carefully documented in the patient's notes. Written information should be provided about contraception, gonadal damage and techniques to preserve fertility. Specialist psychological support and counselling should be available to all these patients.

3   Sperm banking must be considered for all males prior to treatment that carries a risk of long-term gonadal damage. Testicular sperm extraction is sometimes possible even when azoospermia is present. This technique is not currently widely funded.

4   All females should be fully informed at diagnosis of the potential for gonadal or uterine damage caused by anti-cancer treatment, together with the possibility of early menopause.

5   Embryo storage prior to treatment is possible for the minority of patients with a partner and sufficient time for IVF.

6   Egg and ovarian storage are techniques in development which are not currently funded by the National Health Service. Very few live births have been reported after either technique worldwide. It is, however, anticipated that the results will improve. It is recommended that a research-based egg and ovarian tissue storage facility be developed at a number of collaborating sites in the UK, which should be available for younger female patients likely to be sterilised by their cancer treatment.

7   The literature in the field of gonadal toxicity is very limited, with few or no randomised trials. It is imperative that a research base/evidence base be developed in this field. Clinicians are encouraged to seek funding and research bodies to support further studies in this area. In particular the gonadal effects of new anti-cancer agents are very poorly validated.

8   In 2004 the National Institute for Health and Clinical Excellence (NICE) issued a report, *Fertility: assessment and treatment for people with fertility problems*, which considered cryopreservation of gametes and embryos in patients undergoing gonadotoxic treatment. Universal access to sperm, egg and embryo storage was recommended. There is, however, currently no national policy for funding any of the techniques which aim to preserve fertility or treat the effects of gonadal damage, demand for which will always be very limited. The Working Party strongly recommends that an agreed national policy and funded nationwide equity of access to resources be available. Furthermore, we recommend an ongoing audit of the implementation of this recommendation.

9   Provision of sex hormone replacement, where required, should be brought into line with other long-term replacement therapies and be exempt from prescription charges.

Recommendations on funding

NHS funding bodies are strongly encouraged to develop equitable funding protocols for patients in this field, if necessary with national guidance. Access to fertility services is often urgently required when there is a need to proceed quickly with treatment for threatening cancer. The Working Party makes the following recommendations.

1   Long-term sperm banking should be universally available and fully funded. This is a routine evidence-based technique and should be available at short notice to all males commencing treatment which carries any risk of future infertility.

2   Testicular sperm extraction is an established technique for obtaining sperm for IVF in patients who are azoospermic either before or after treatment with chemotherapy. The Working Party recommends that this procedure be available nationwide to appropriately selected males.

3   A small minority of females with cancer who require chemotherapy or irradiation likely to cause infertility are suitable for emergency IVF (implying egg harvesting and IVF using a partner's sperm). It is strongly recommended that this service be provided at short notice for appropriate female patients likely to be sterilised by their treatment. It is accepted that this may give patients with cancer precedence over those seeking treatment for infertility in other circumstances.

4   Egg and ovarian tissue storage techniques should currently be regarded as developmental. These are not at present widely available with NHS funding but are often provided in the private sector. National funding bodies (Cancer Research UK, the Medical Research Council and Department of Health) are strongly encouraged to fund development of a small network of research-based centres providing universal access to and further development of these techniques. It is anticipated that the technology in this field will rapidly improve in the next few years. An evidence-based approach to the management of the small minority of patients requiring these techniques is essential.

5   There is no routine NHS provision for manipulation of stored gametes or embryos once cancer treatment has been completed. This is regarded as inappropriate and routine funding streams should be available for these patients.

6   Male and female hormone replacement treatments are currently not exempt from prescription charges. This is anomalous given the national funding arrangements for other endocrine replacement treatments. It is recommended that these treatments be exempt from prescription charges.

7   Psychosocial support independent of treating clinicians should be routinely available and funded for all patients described in this report.

Abbreviations

AIH	Artificial insemination by husband's/partner's semen
ALL	Acute lymphoblastic leukaemia
AMH	Anti-Mullerian hormone
AML	Acute myeloid leukaemia
BMT	Bone marrow transplant
CIS	Carcinoma *in situ*
DH	Department of Health
EORTC	European Organisation for Research and Treatment of Cancer
FSH	Follicle-stimulating hormone
GTD	Gestational trophoblastic disease
Gy	Gray – a unit of radiotherapy dose
HCG	Human chorionic gonadotrophin
HFEA	Human Fertility and Embryology Authority
HIV	Human immunodeficiency virus
HL	Hodgkin lymphoma
HRT	Hormone replacement therapy
HTA	Human Tissue Authority
ICSI	Intracytoplasmic sperm injection
IVF	*In vitro* fertilisation
IVM	*In vitro* maturation
LH	Luteinising hormone
LHRH	Luteinising hormone releasing hormone
LNG	Levonorgestrel
MRC	Medical Research Council
MRI	Magnetic resonance imaging
NHL	Non-Hodgkin lymphoma
NICE	National Institute for Health and Clinical Excellence
PSA	Prostate-specific antigen
RCOG	Royal College of Obstetricians and Gynaecologists
RCP	Royal College of Physicians
RCR	Royal College of Radiologists
RT	Radiotherapy
SHBG	Sex hormone binding globulin

SSRI	Selective serotonin releasing inhibitor
TBI	Total body irradiation
TSR	Testicular sperm retrieval

Chemotherapy regimens

ABVD	Adriamycin (doxorubicin), bleomycin, vinblastine and dacarbazine
BEACOPP	Bleomycin, etoposide, Adriamycin (doxorubicin), cyclophosphamide, Oncovin (vincristine), procarbazine and prednisolone
BEAM	BCNU (carmustine), etoposide, ara-c (cytarabine) and melphalan
BEP	Bleomycin, etoposide and platinum (cisplatin)
CHOP	Cyclophosphamide, hydroxydaunomycin (doxorubicin), Oncovin (vincristine) and prednisolone
CODOX-M/IVAC	Cyclophosphamide, Oncovin (vincristine), doxorubicin, methotrexate, ifosfamide, mesna, etoposide (VP-16) and cytarabine (ara-c)
DHAP	Dexamethasone, high-dose ara-c (cytarabine) and platinum (cisplatin)
ESHAP	Etoposide, steroid (methyl prednisolone), high-dose ara-c (cytarabine) and platinum (cisplatin)
ICE	Ifosfamide, carboplatin and etoposide
R-CHOP	Rituximab, cyclophosphamide, hydroxydaunomycin (doxorubicin), Oncovin (vincristine) and prednisolone
R-CVP	Rituximab, cyclophosphamide, Oncovin (vincristine) and prednisolone
VAPEC-B	Vincristine, Adriamycin (doxorubicin), prednisolone, etoposide, cyclophosphamide and bleomycin

1 Introduction

1.1 This report is the work of a multidisciplinary expert group. Members of the group examined the current literature describing gonadal toxicity in relation to cancer treatment, including current reviews and a consensus document.[1,2] The literature in this area is relatively sparse, mainly comprising case studies, with very few randomised trials. In view of this, the report predominantly comprises expert consensus or guidance rather than a formal evidence-based approach. It should be noted that chemotherapy drugs are also used to treat benign diseases. The comments in this document apply also to groups treated in this way.

1.2 Many techniques for fertility preservation are currently unavailable or infrequently available to National Health Service (NHS) patients. It is hoped that this report will encourage funding (in some cases research-based) of some of the new developments described, on an equitable basis. In this regard we have produced advice to funding bodies about possible allocation of resources in this important area (p x).

Background

1.3 Cancer affects over 11,000 patients per year in the UK in the 15–40 years age group, comprising 4% of patients with cancer.[3] A diagnosis of cancer has a devastating impact on patients and their families in this age group. Although cure of the cancer is of paramount importance, the effect of the disease on fertility at the time of presentation and of the potential gonadal damage caused by treatment with surgery, chemotherapy or radiotherapy must also be considered.

1.4 In 1998 the Royal College of Physicians (RCP) and Royal College of Radiologists (RCR) produced a joint report entitled *Management of gonadal toxicity resulting from the treatment of adult cancer.*[4] The report identified gonadal damage in young adults resulting from cancer treatment, and provided cross-disciplinary advice about appropriate management. The current report updates that report, as much has changed. Multiple new chemotherapy agents, small molecules and antibodies are now in routine use alone and in combination, often with uncertain or unknown gonadal effects. In addition, the management of anticipated gonadal damage and infertility has also changed, although many of the new advances are either unavailable or inconsistently available to NHS patients. For example, new possibilities for ovarian tissue storage are widely described, but seldom actually available.

1.5 Patient demands for information, support and, where necessary, treatment continue to increase, but are often not adequately met.

1.6 In this report we describe normal human reproduction physiology, the potential damaging effects of anti-cancer drugs and irradiation, and techniques available to prevent, ameliorate, or manage consequent damage.

2 Reproductive physiology

Fertility in males

2.1   Sperm production in males is maintained by production of follicle-stimulating hormone (FSH) by the pituitary gland, regulated by a negative feedback mechanism by inhibin produced from the seminiferous tubules within the testis. Androgen production is maintained by pituitary production of luteinising hormone (LH) also controlled by a negative feedback mechanism by production of testosterone by the testicular Leydig cells.

2.2   Mature sperm are produced in the testis and travel along the epididymis to be stored in the vas deferens. Sperm are not fertile when they leave the testes (unless manipulated *in vitro*, eg by intracytoplasmic sperm injection (ICSI)). They acquire fertilising capacity as they pass along the epididymis.

2.3   Fertility is most effectively assessed by a semen analysis, with the assessment of sperm concentration, motility and percentage of normal forms. 'Normal' values[5] are:

▶   sperm concentration $>20 \times 10^6$/ml

▶   >50% of sperm motile

▶   >14% normal forms (this figure is controversial but acceptable as a guide).

It should be noted that if *in vitro* fertilisation (IVF) – particularly ICSI – techniques are used, men with very low sperm counts such as $<1 \times 10^6$/ml are potentially fertile. FSH levels provide a less accurate means of assessing sperm production. Elevated levels are associated with reduced (or absent) spermatogenesis.

2.4   Sperm can be retrieved from the epididymis or from the testis and can be used to inject eggs. These techniques are very successful, resulting in live birth rates in an average of 15% of cycles started.[6] In the UK, regulation dictates that only mature sperm can be injected into an egg. Immature sperm (spermatids) cannot be used in treatment.

Fertility in females

2.5   In normally menstruating women, ovarian function depends primarily on pituitary production of LH and FSH. FSH stimulates the granulosa cells of the growing follicle to proliferate and produce oestradiol. This causes feedback inhibition of the pituitary, maintaining FSH at a low level. Ovulation occurs in response to the midcycle LH surge, following which the corpus luteum produces progesterone.

2.6   Follicle development, from the resting primordial stage until ovulation, takes several months. In addition to oestradiol, growing follicles also produce peptide hormones, which are also important in feedback regulation of FSH. Inhibin B is produced by small follicles and therefore highest levels are measured during the early follicular phase. Inhibin A levels rise in the later follicular phase and reflect development of the dominant follicle.

2.7   At puberty, approximately 200,000 ovarian follicles are present in the ovary. This number progressively declines with age, with accelerated loss after age 35, to a few hundred at the time of menopause. In younger women the larger number of follicles and therefore higher inhibin B concentrations result in lower FSH concentrations. FSH is most accurately determined in the early follicular phase before emergence of a dominant follicle, ie days 1–5 following onset of menses. As women age the number of follicles in the ovary falls, and there is a reduction in feedback inhibition so circulating FSH levels rise.

2.8   The number of follicles in the ovary determines the remaining 'reproductive lifespan'. This is known as the ovarian reserve. In addition to FSH and inhibin B discussed above, anti-Mullerian hormone (AMH) is emerging as a promising measure of the ovarian reserve,[7] but the latter two tests are only available at present in a research context. AMH is produced by follicles as soon as they start to grow, but declines when the follicle becomes 'antral', ie contains a fluid cavity and becomes FSH-dependent. Production of AMH is therefore from smaller less mature follicles than inhibin and oestradiol and has the advantage of little variability across the menstrual cycle (Fig 1). Ultrasound measures of ovarian volume and antral follicle counts can also be used to assess the size of the ovarian reserve. Older women with a smaller ovarian reserve are more likely to become menopausal following treatment for cancer with a given chemotherapy regimen than younger women.

2.9   Regular menstruation and ovulation can be maintained in the presence of a severely depleted ovarian reserve, ie until shortly before the menopause, and should not be taken as an indication of normal fertility. Persisting amenorrhoea with an FSH level greater than 30 IU/I implies onset of the menopause. Approximately 1% of women in the UK will have a menopause before the age of 40. The median age is 51 years.

2.10   Spontaneous regular menses imply ovulatory cycles, and potential fertility can occasionally recover after cancer treatment, in some cases after many months or years. In some this will be short-lived, but this may allow a window for conception, particularly in younger women.

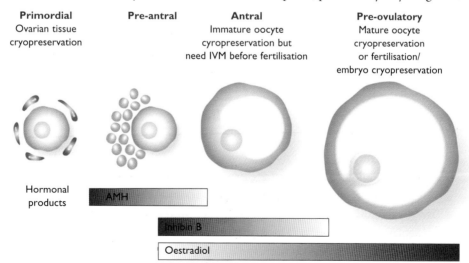

Fig 1. Diagram illustrating changing patterns of hormone production by ovarian follicles as they develop from the resting, primordial stage through pre-antral and antral to pre-ovulatory stages. Darker shading in hormone labels corresponds to greater hormone production. The text indicates possible techniques for fertility preservation (see sections 5.19 et seq). AMH = anti-Mullerian hormone; IVM = *in vitro* maturation.

3 Effects of cancer treatment on fertility

Gonadal effects of chemotherapy

Males

3.1   Chemotherapy can directly damage spermatogenesis temporarily or permanently, but androgen production by the testis is usually much less affected.

3.2   The degree of gonadal stem cell damage varies according to the drugs used, dose, route of administration (oral *v* intravenous), treatment regimen (eg combination therapies) and total doses of individual chemotherapeutic agents.[2] It is probable, although not well documented, that this also relates to pre-treatment sperm counts.

3.3   It is clear and well documented that the most toxic drugs are the alkylating agents, and that their use can cause permanent azoospermia. Limited or no data exist for many of the newer agents and the working assumption may be that these are also gonadotoxic. It is important that a research base/evidence base be developed in this area, perhaps coupled with clinical trials. Clinicians and research bodies are encouraged to support such studies.

3.4   Low sperm counts or azoospermia are common after treatment of patients with combination chemotherapy regimes. Recovery can occur subject to the above conditions, but may take years. Data about individual treatment regimens used in younger patients will be given in the appropriate treatment-related sections.

Females

3.5   The ovary is chemo-sensitive. Chemotherapy can result in loss of primordial and growing follicles, with consequent loss of hormone production and menstruation, and an early menopause. Ovarian toxicity varies depending on the regimen, therefore the result will vary from no apparent effect, through incomplete loss of follicles resulting in an early menopause, to rapid and permanent ovarian failure. Some drugs, particularly alkylating agents, are more damaging to the ovary than other agents[8] but there are very limited data quantifying the extent of ovarian damage.[9]

3.6   The impact of combination cytotoxic chemotherapy on gonadal function is dependent on the nature and total dosage of the drugs administered and is very strongly influenced by the age of patient. Younger women have more oocytes and as a consequence gonadal toxicity may appear less severe than in older women, since their ovaries still support regular ovarian cycles despite a depleted oocyte reserve. The symptoms associated with the menopausal transition are irregular menstrual cycles, vasomotor (hot flushes, night sweats) and urogenital changes (urinary frequency, urgency, vaginal dryness and superficial dyspareunia).

3.7   New chemotherapeutic drugs in multi-agent chemotherapy protocols need to be continuously evaluated to determine the risk of late effects including ovarian failure.

Gonadal effects of irradiation

Males

3.8   The testes are directly irradiated in the treatment of leukaemic relapse, tumours of the lower pelvis and carcinoma *in situ* (CIS) of the testis. The germinal epithelium is highly sensitive to irradiation and unlike most tissues is not spared by fractionation. The threshold dose for effect is low, and with increasing dose there is a rapid increase in damage. The degree of risk will be dose- and technique-dependent.

3.9   Transient suppression with subsequent recovery of spermatogenesis occurs with doses as low as 0.5 Gy. Following 2–3 Gy there is a period of azoospermia after which full recovery is expected within three years; at doses of 4–6 Gy recovery is not universal and may take up to five years; after 6 Gy there is a high risk of permanent sterility. Total body irradiation (TBI) with high-dose chemotherapy will sterilise men.[10]

3.10   The Leydig cell is more resistant to irradiation. Nevertheless, a dose of irradiation in excess of 15 Gy may be sufficient to affect Leydig cell function and production of testosterone, and a dose of 24 Gy will irreversibly damage the Leydig cells in prepubertal boys.

3.11   When directly in the irradiation field the testes cannot be protected. The dose from scattered irradiation from nearby beams can, however, be reduced by moving the gonad away from the beam and, in some circumstances, by applying thick shielding cups directly over the scrotum. Displacement of the scrotum away from lateral pelvic and proximal thigh fields with taping during radiotherapy may be the most effective means available.

3.12   The beneficial effect of specific testicular shielding in reducing the dose from scattered irradiation has been debated and depends on the position and nature of the radiation field. Irradiation to the pelvic lymph node areas, as in the treatment of testicular tumours or lymphoma, results in a scattered dose to the testis of 1.5–3 Gy. In this situation, testicular shielding may be used and the dose reduced to the order of 0.5–0.8 Gy.[11,12] Shielding placed directly on and around the scrotum is required and needs to be of a thickness to reduce an incident dose to 5% or less. The practical difficulties of this are considerable and the shield may impede the more effective measure of displacing the scrotum away from the beam, as described above.

Females

Ovary

3.13   The ovaries are within or close to the irradiation field in the treatment of gynaecological malignancies and in tumours of the pelvic bones, soft tissue and lymph nodes within the pelvis and the proximal thigh.

3.14   Irradiation produces severe dose-related gonadal damage to both the germ cell and endocrine components of ovarian tissue. It may cause immediate permanent sterility, temporary cessation of menses or lead to a premature menopause. The probability of infertility from a given dose of radiotherapy increases with age and concurrent use of chemotherapy: immediate ovarian failure will be produced by 16.5 Gy in females of 20 years, while 14 Gy is sufficient in 30-year-olds.[13]

3.15   If the ovaries are adjacent to irradiation beams but not in the target volume, the dose can be minimised by the use of adequate shielding, by angulation of the treatment head or by a nondivergent border adjacent to the ovary in question. However, the level of scattered irradiation may still be sufficient to destroy function in this ovary and methods of oophoropexy (surgical relocation of the ovary) should be considered.[14]

Uterus

3.16   Partial uterine radiation may occur in treatment of the pelvic lymph nodes, rectal cancer or sarcomas of the pelvic side walls. Whole uterine radiotherapy occurs in treatment of gynaecological tumours, anal and central pelvic sarcomas.

3.17   The reported effects of radiotherapy may be complicated by the effects of oestrogen deficiency. Endometrial function, in terms of cyclical changes, may be maintained after exposure to doses as high as 40 Gy. There will, however, be a risk of vascular insufficiency and fibrosis. After uterine irradiation, magnetic resonance imaging (MRI) appearances resemble those of a non-irradiated postmenopausal uterus. Irradiation doses of 20–30 Gy to the uterus result in an increased rate of miscarriage. Pregnancy may occur after relatively low doses of radiation, as in treatments for dysgerminoma or TBI and where parametrial radiation produces partial uterine radiotherapy.[15,16]

Hypothalamic–pituitary irradiation

3.18   Irradiation to the hypothalamic–pituitary axis may produce deficiencies in gonadotrophin production. This will be manifest as amenorrhoea/hypogonadotrophic hypogonadism many years later and is more likely to occur when pituitary reserve is already diminished (as by pituitary tumour surgery). Doses of 45 Gy in adults, but less in children (24–35 Gy) carry significant risk of deficiency. Such doses may be administered in cranial prophylaxis for leukaemia, brain tumours and tumours of the orbit and paranasal sinuses.

Total body irradiation

3.19   Total body irradiation (TBI) is likely to result in ovarian failure.[17] Young women exposed to TBI may exhibit impaired uterine growth and blood flow, and uterine volume may be reduced by as much as 40% of normal adult values. Young women or children treated with TBI and high-dose chemotherapy need to appreciate that if a pregnancy is achieved, either with a spontaneous conception or ovum donation, there is an increased risk of early pregnancy loss, growth retardation and pre-term birth.

Radioisotope therapy

3.20   Radioactive iodine treatment for cancer causes no increase in infertility, miscarriage, prematurity or congenital abnormalities from the protocols used in most patients, whether male or female.[18–20] The irradiation dose to the gonads is dependent on the iodine uptake by the thyroid and also the dose from the iodine secreted in the bladder. The patient should maintain a high fluid intake and void the bladder frequently after receiving treatment. Transient amenorrhoea may occur. The general advice is to avoid pregnancy for one year after the administration of the radioactive isotope. While there is no good evidence of an adverse effect, it is a sensible precaution[21] to offer sperm storage to those men likely to require several doses of radioiodine.

4   Effects of treatment of specific cancers on fertility

Introduction

4.1   These sections provide more detailed information about management approaches and gonadal toxicity in the malignancies that are most common in patients of reproductive age. A number of issues recur in each section.

4.2   It is important that all patients are advised of the treatment options available for their cancer, some of which may be associated with less gonadal toxicity. A written record should be maintained of this discussion and of any decisions about gamete storage. It should be emphasised that adequate contraception is essential during and following chemotherapy, hormonal therapy or irradiation likely to involve the gametes. Information leaflets (eg those provided in Appendix 2) should be provided to all patients.

4.3   Sperm for banking is best obtained prior to initial chemotherapy as this will commonly result in oligo/azoospermia of varying duration. Banking may then be impossible if early relapse occurs. In many cancers such a relapse will be treated with highly gonadotoxic treatment causing sterility. Similar considerations apply to females; however, the techniques of egg/ovarian strip storage (see sections 5.22–5.26) are not currently widely available or funded and may take time. In such cases, deferment of such storage, when agreed, may best be made to the time of relapse, should it occur.

4.4   Malignancies sometimes spread to the gonads. This risk is greatest with the leukaemias and Burkitt's lymphoma, but should be considered in all patients with metastatic disease. Such involvement may still allow sperm and possibly even egg/embryo cryopreservation. Reimplantation of cryopreserved gonadal tissue would clearly be inappropriate, but future developments may allow *in vitro* maturation or the use of animal xenografting, which at present are not possible.

Breast cancer

Introduction

4.5   Over 90% of women present with disease localised to the breast which, with appropriate local and systemic therapies, can be successfully managed with a high probability of long-term survival. Around 70% of women presenting with early breast cancer can now expect to be alive without evidence of breast cancer at 10 years.[22]

Management

Early stage of the disease

4.6   Management of the early stage of breast cancer relies on multidisciplinary care with high-quality surgery and radiotherapy to optimise local control, and appropriate use of adjuvant systemic treatments. For women with oestrogen-responsive tumours endocrine treatments are routinely used, while chemotherapy is recommended for patients at moderate to high risk of recurrence, especially in premenopausal women and for tumours lacking oestrogen receptors.[23,24] Trastuzumab is an antibody to the HER2 growth factor receptor expressed by 20–25% of breast cancers and is also now used in the adjuvant setting.[25]

Metastatic disease

4.7   Treatment of metastatic breast cancer is palliative with a median survival of two years. Endocrine treatments, chemotherapy, trastuzumab and palliative radiotherapy all have a role in maintaining disease control and quality of life for as long as possible.

Chemotherapy

4.8   Adjuvant chemotherapy is increasingly used in the management of breast cancer and modern regimens reduce the annual risks of recurrence and death by 30–40% and 20–30% respectively.[22] In premenopausal women chemotherapy may induce a premature menopause. This becomes more likely with increasing age, and with regimens containing an alkylating agent such as cyclophosphamide.[26] Approximately 30–50% of women who receive chemotherapy in their 30s and 50–100% of those treated in their 40s will experience a premature menopause and be rendered infertile. Chemotherapy-induced ovarian suppression may be temporary in some women (especially those who are younger) with recovery of menstrual function occurring months to several years after completion of chemotherapy. However, even when menstrual function is maintained or recovers, the menopause usually occurs earlier than expected on average by 5–10 years.[27, 28]

4.9   Strategies to reduce the risks of chemotherapy-induced menopause include avoidance of alkylating drugs from the regimen and the use of LHRH (luteinising hormone releasing hormone) analogues to suppress ovarian function and possibly protect against long-term damage. Case series suggest the latter approach may be useful, but definitive proof awaits the results of ongoing randomised trials.[29] For women who wish to retain the possibility of future fertility, urgent referral to a specialist infertility service is recommended to discuss the available options including embryo and egg storage (see sections 5.19–5.26). Delay of adjuvant chemotherapy for 1–2 menstrual cycles may be clinically acceptable while ovarian stimulation and egg harvesting take place. Close links and regular discussion between the oncologist and reproductive medicine service are essential.[30]

Adjuvant endocrine therapy

4.10   Breast cancer that is potentially oestrogen-responsive is identified by immunohistochemical detection of oestrogen receptors on the primary tumour. In this setting, endocrine treatment reduces the annual risks of recurrence and death by 40–50% and 25–30% respectively.[22]

4.11   In premenopausal women, ovarian suppression or ablation plus tamoxifen (which is not contraceptive) for five years is the preferred treatment. For women wishing to retain fertility, ovarian suppression with an LHRH analogue for at least two years is recommended.[23] Ovarian function usually recovers over 3–12 months after stopping the LHRH analogue. Tamoxifen may be used on its own in premenopausal women. Although it may result in menstrual irregularity it does not adversely affect fertility.[31]

Management of menopausal symptoms

4.12   Many thousands of women with breast cancer experience a premature menopause as a result of adjuvant chemotherapy and endocrine treatments. Additionally, tamoxifen and the aromatase inhibitors typically exacerbate the vasomotor symptoms of the menopause. Treatment of these symptoms is difficult. Hormone replacement therapy (HRT) is generally contraindicated, especially in the context of a hormone-sensitive tumour. Patients often use various herbal remedies and dietary supplements. The ingredients should be checked as some contain oestrogenic compounds.[32] Recent reviews have questioned the real benefit of these adjunct supplements to provide symptom benefit.[33] Pharmacological management of vasomotor symptoms with clonidine and the selective serotonin-releasing inhibitors (SSRIs), such as venlafaxine and paroxetine, may be useful. Alternative endocrine agents such as medroxyprogesterone acetate and tibolone[34] are occasionally used and a large randomised trial (Liberate) assessing the safety of tibolone in breast cancer survivors has recently completed accrual with outcome data awaited.

Pregnancy after breast cancer

4.13   Women who have completed adjuvant treatment for early breast cancer may wish to start or resume having a family. It has been typical practice to encourage a delay of 2–3 years after a diagnosis of breast cancer to ensure that any potential risks to the fetus from chemotherapy exposure have been minimised. Delay also allows the peak incidence for breast cancer recurrence to pass although, unlike most other malignancies, late recurrence of breast cancer is relatively common with an annual risk of around 2–3% up to 10 years and 1–2% up to 15 years. Although the evidence available is confined to case series and epidemiological studies, pregnancy after breast cancer does not appear to affect cancer outcome adversely, irrespective of the endocrine sensitivity of the previous tumour.[35] Recent data suggest that prolonged delay may not be necessary, with favourable outcomes in terms of both the pregnancy and the probability of breast cancer recurrence in women who become pregnant at least six months after diagnosis.[36] It remains recommended, however, to delay conception for a year after chemotherapy because of possible mutagenic effects on the oocyte, although this is not based on good evidence.

Hodgkin and non-Hodgkin lymphoma

Introduction

4.14   A significant number of patients with lymphoma can look forward to prolonged survival and for this reason the impact of treatment on fertility is of great relevance. This is particularly the case for those with Hodgkin lymphoma (HL) where the median age at diagnosis is in the region of 30 years and where approximately 70% will be cured as a result of first or second-line treatment. Non-Hodgkin lymphomas (NHL) occur in an older population (median age at presentation, 60 years) but NHL is more common than HL and a significant number of patients with NHL will be younger men or women with concerns about future fertility. Hodgkin lymphoma, particularly when advanced, is associated with infertility and low sperm counts in males. Recovery generally occurs if non-gonadotoxic chemotherapy is used (eg Adriamycin (doxorubicin), bleomycin, vinblastine and dacarbazine (ABVD); see below).

Hodgkin lymphoma

First-line treatment of stages IA and IIA

4.15   Cure rates are very high. Wide-field irradiation using mantle or inverted Y fields for early stage disease has now been superseded by abbreviated chemotherapy followed by involved field radiotherapy. Unless the radiotherapy (RT) field employed is sub-diaphragmatic, both male and female fertility are unlikely to be affected by treatment of this type. Nonetheless sperm banking (see sections 5.4–5.10) is recommended and egg/ovarian storage should at least be discussed (see sections 5.19–5.26). Patients can, however, be reassured that no intervention may be necessary to support future fertility.

First-line treatment of stages IB, IIB, III and IV

4.16   For some years the international standard of care for these stages has been 6–8 cycles ABVD followed by RT to sites of initial bulk and/or residual radiographic abnormality. There remains interest in the intensification of treatment for the minority of patients with high-risk disease (Hasenclever score ≥5) and a randomised trial by the European Organisation for Research and Treatment of Cancer (EORTC) comparing ABVD with escalated BEACOPP (bleomycin, etoposide, Adriamycin (doxorubicin), cyclophosphamide, Oncovin (vincristine), procarbazine and prednisolone) (see section 4.18) is underway.

4.17   Depending on the number of cycles administered, ABVD is associated with temporary oligozoospermia/azoospermia, but recovery of the sperm count usually occurs by 18 months. Nevertheless, semen analysis and storage (sections 5.4–5.10) should be offered as a routine against the possibility of no recovery or of relapse requiring gonadotoxic treatment. Amenorrhoea is common, but unless the woman is over the age of 40 this is very unlikely to be permanent and no active intervention is generally necessary to support future fertility.

4.18   BEACOPP is substantially more toxic than ABVD and although published data are not yet available, permanent azoospermia is likely and, depending on the age of the patient, so too is permanent amenorrhoea. For these patients, semen storage for men (sections 5.4–5.10) and embryo/egg/ovarian tissue storage for women (sections 5.19–5.26) should be considered in all cases before treatment.

Salvage treatment

4.19   For the shrinking pool of patients previously treated with RT alone who later relapse, ABVD is likely to be the treatment offered (see section 4.17). For patients relapsing after combined modality treatment, re-induction chemotherapy followed at remission by high-dose BEAM (BCNU (carmustine), etoposide, ara-c (cytarabine) and melphalan) with autologous haematopoietic stem cell rescue will probably be recommended for younger patients and therefore permanent infertility is likely. Although there are anecdotal reports of recovery of fertility in both sexes, semen storage for men (sections 5.4–5.10) and embryo/egg/ovarian tissue storage for women (sections 5.19–5.26) should be considered in all cases.

Non-Hodgkin lymphoma

4.20   The many different sub-types of NHL are managed in different ways, from the watch-and-wait policy where there is clearly no effect on gonadal function to the very intensive CODOX–M/IVAC schedule for Burkitt's lymphoma. In between these two extremes is a large cohort of patients with symptomatic or large-volume follicular lymphoma and diffuse large B-cell lymphoma, all of whom require treatment with moderately intensive regimens. In recent years the monoclonal antibody rituximab has revolutionised the treatment of B-cell lymphomas and although sometimes given alone (where there is likely to be no impact on gonadal function) this agent is now usually given in combination with chemotherapy.

First-line treatment of indolent sub-types of NHL

4.21   A watch-and-wait policy is likely to be recommended for patients with asymptomatic, low-volume disease, but for the majority treatment will be required. In the minority of individuals with stages IA/IIA, local RT can be curative and unless disease has a pelvic presentation, there will be no impact on gonadal function.

4.22   In the more usual situation of symptomatic and/or bulky stages III or IV disease, first-line treatment with 6–8 cycles of R-CVP (rituximab, cyclophosphamide, vincristine (Oncovin) and prednisolone) or R-CHOP (rituximab, cyclophosphamide, hydroxydaunomycin (doxorubicin), vincristine (Oncovin) and prednisolone) is likely to be recommended and permanent azoospermia/amenorrhoea is possible. Although the latter is rare in women treated under the age of 40, semen storage for men (sections 5.4–5.10) and embryo/egg/ovarian tissue storage for women (sections 5.19–5.26) should be considered in all cases.

Second and subsequent treatment for indolent sub-types

4.23   Re-induction chemotherapy followed at remission by high-dose BEAM with autologous haematopoietic stem cell rescue is likely to be recommended for younger patients and allogeneic bone marrow transplantation may also be considered in high-risk disease. Although there are anecdotal reports of recovery of fertility in both sexes, there is a high risk of permanent infertility, and unless semen storage for men (sections 5.4–5.10) and embryo/egg/ovarian tissue storage for women (sections 5.19–5.26) has already been arranged these should be considered in all cases.

4.24   For older patients or those not wishing to receive high-dose chemotherapy other options include fludarabine-containing therapies and radioimmunotherapy but there are few data on the gonadal effects of these treatments.

First-line treatment of aggressive sub-types

4.25   For patients with low-risk stage I diffuse large B cell lymphoma, three cycles of CHOP followed by involved field RT is recommended, but for those with high-risk, stage I disease 6–8 cycles of R-CHOP may be preferred. The latter is standard care for stages II–IV and permanent azoospermia/amenorrhoea is possible. Although permanent amenorrhoea is rare in women treated under the age of 40, semen storage for men (sections 5.4–5.10) and embryo/egg/ovarian tissue storage for women (sections 5.19–5.26) should be considered in all cases if the patient is fit enough for this to be undertaken.

4.26   In Burkitt's lymphoma, three cycles of CODOX-M (for low-risk disease) or two cycles of CODOX-M alternating with two cycles of IVAC (for high-risk disease) could produce permanent azoospermia, and women are at significant risk of permanent amenorrhoea. Semen storage for men (sections 5.4–5.10) and embryo/egg/ovarian tissue storage for women (sections 5.19–5.23) should be considered in all cases if the patient is fit enough for this to be undertaken. It should, however, be noted that this lymphoma can spread to the ovaries in women with advanced disease.

Second-line treatment for aggressive sub-types

4.27   For younger and fitter patients, re-induction chemotherapy with the platinum-containing DHAP (dexamethasone, high-dose ara-c (cytarabine) and platinum (cisplatin)), ICE (ifosfamide, carboplatin and etoposide) or ESHAP (etoposide, steroid (methyl prednisolone), high-dose ara-c (cytarabine) and platinum (cisplatin)) regimens followed at remission by high-dose BEAM with autologous haematopoietic stem cell rescue is likely to be recommended. These treatments following R-CHOP are highly damaging to gonadal function although anecdotally recovery does sometimes occur. In most cases, semen will have previously been cryopreserved, but for women gamete storage may not have been arranged and this should therefore be discussed (sections 5.19–5.26).

Testicular cancer

Introduction

4.28   Germ cell cancer of the testis occurs at a median age of 30 years and fertility is a common issue in the management of these patients. These cancers are sometimes associated with reduced fertility and androgen production before, and particularly after treatment by orchidectomy.[37] Additional treatment with irradiation or chemotherapy will increase these risks.[38,39] Progressive testicular failure can occur even in the absence of treatment, and may relate in some cases to the presence of contralateral carcinoma *in situ*.[40]

4.29   Irradiation is now used infrequently in the management of germ cell cancer and its use is almost confined to early stage seminoma or carcinoma *in situ* of the testis. Patients with stage I seminoma can be adequately managed with para-aortic irradiation (20 Gy)[41] and stage IIA/B with para-aortic and iliac dog-leg irradiation (30 Gy). Carcinoma *in situ* is usually treated with 20 Gy to the testis.[42]

4.30   Chemotherapy is used as part of the management of most patients with germ cell cancer. The most common regimens are single agent carboplatin for stage I seminoma[43] and BEP (bleomycin, etoposide and platinum (cisplatin)) used as an adjuvant for high-risk teratoma (two cycles) or for advanced teratoma or seminoma (three or four cycles).

Management

4.31   In clinical practice, oncologists are first involved with non-metastatic testis cancer after orchidectomy. Surgeons should, however, be aware that pre-orchidectomy sperm banking may be preferable if the non-tumour-bearing testis is small and potentially non-functioning.[37] FSH/LH and testosterone levels should be evaluated routinely after orchidectomy and repeated as indicated after treatment. FSH and LH levels are often temporarily suppressed in the presence of elevated HCG (human chorionic gonadotrophin).

Surveillance for stage I disease

4.32　Sperm banking is not routinely recommended. Evaluation of FSH, LH and testosterone levels should be repeated as relevant if they were initially abnormal. Occasionally hormone replacement therapy (HRT) will be required. Sperm banking should be considered if there is a risk of testicular failure (see sections 5.4-5.10).

Contralateral testicular biopsy

4.33　A sperm count and storage should be offered prior to this procedure. Carcinoma *in situ* is often associated with low or absent sperm in the ejaculate,[44] so testicular sperm retrieval (TSR) (see section 5.11) may be considered where relevant at the time of biopsy in this circumstance.

Radiotherapy

4.34　Para-aortic irradiation should not affect gonadal function and sperm banking is therefore unnecessary.[41]

4.35　Dog-leg irradiation (using shielding) will cause only transient lowering of sperm counts, although cancer relapse, if it occurs, would require potentially sterilising chemotherapy. Sperm banking is therefore generally indicated where relevant[41] (sections 5.4–5.10).

4.36　Testicular irradiation for CIS results in permanent infertility with a significant risk of hypogonadism which increases with time.[42] Sperm banking or TSR, as appropriate (sections 5.4–5.11), should be considered before irradiation. Sequential LH and testosterone levels should be measured after treatment.

Chemotherapy

4.37　A small proportion of patients present with gross advanced metastatic cancer. In this case sperm banking may not be possible or can take place on only one occasion. Patients requiring post-chemotherapy retroperitoneal lymphadenectomy may, unusually, develop retrograde ejaculation and should be advised of this possibility.

4.38　Neither carboplatin[43] nor bleomycin, etoposide and platinum (cisplatin) (2–4 cycles)[39] will cause long-term infertility in the great majority of patients. However, patients with low initial sperm counts may require years to recover, and when second-line or subsequent chemotherapy (or post-chemotherapy retroperitoneal surgery) is required, recovery may not occur. Sperm banking (sections 5.4–5.10) is therefore recommended before chemotherapy where relevant. If no sperm is present in the ejaculate, and metastatic disease is non-threatening, TSR may be considered.

4.39　Sperm counts normally recover 1–5 years after chemotherapy and banked sperm is not usually needed. Where recovery is poor, banked sperm can be used for IVF or intracytoplasmic sperm injection (ICSI) as appropriate (sections 6.11–6.13), or TSR (section 5.11) can be considered where sperm was not banked.[45]

4.40　FSH and, to a lesser extent, LH levels are commonly elevated after chemotherapy and decrease with time. Long-term studies show ongoing minor elevation of LH levels, with slight reduction of testosterone as a common late effect.[46] In a small proportion of patients, overt hypogonadism will occur and require lifelong testosterone replacement. The management of more marginal biochemical clinical cases needs to be individualised (see sections 8.7–8.17).

Cervical cancer

Introduction

4.41   Carcinoma of the cervix is the second most common malignancy in UK women under 35, with the highest incidence between the ages of 30 and 45. Over the past 25 years the overall incidence of cervical cancer has decreased but so has the age at diagnosis.[47] These demographic changes, together with the trend to delay first pregnancy, have resulted in significant numbers of younger women needing treatment yet wishing to retain fertility. For those with small-volume disease confined to the cervix, a less radical surgical approach might be possible. Where cure will not be compromised, the ovaries are conserved as is, in highly selected cases, the body of the uterus.

Standard radical treatment

4.42   For more advanced disease, the standard treatment with radical (curative intent) surgery or radiotherapy to the cervix is necessary, but this inevitably destroys uterine function. Radical surgery removes the uterus, ovaries and tubes together with the draining lymph nodes and upper vagina. Radical radiotherapy treats the pelvis using a combination of high energy X-rays (external beam radiotherapy) and a temporarily placed intrauterine radioactive source (brachytherapy). After pelvic radiotherapy ovarian failure will be rapid and the uterus will become non-distensible with gradual loss of cellular structure and the development of fibrosis. These patients are not expected to have ovarian function or to be able to carry a pregnancy.

Early disease: conservation of the ovaries

4.43   When the cancer is confined to the cervix it may be possible to conserve the ovaries, surgically removing only the uterus and draining lymph nodes. In this way egg and ovarian hormone production is retained, but without a uterus the ability to support a pregnancy is lost. However, surrogacy using the patient's own eggs would be possible (see sections 7.1–7.3).

4.44   When external beam radiation treatment to the pelvis is essential, this will usually destroy ovarian function. Surgical mobilisation and fixation of an ovary in the paracolic gutter at the pelvic sidewall (oophoropexy) can be considered.[48] However, vascular damage to the ovary can occur, and the radiation dose may not be reduced sufficiently to prevent sterility.

Very early disease: trachelectomy

4.45   In young women with small (max 2 cm) tumours confined to the cervix, vaginal 'cervicectomy' or 'trachelectomy' (Greek *trachelos* = neck) might enable some women to retain fertility and carry a pregnancy. These cases are carefully selected, usually after laparoscopic lymphadenectomy has demonstrated negative nodes. The operation involves removal of the cervix and upper part of the vagina, leaving behind the body of the uterus while a drawn thread stitch takes the place of the cervix.[49] Spontaneous pregnancies have occurred after trachelectomy, some with a successful outcome but there is a substantial increased risk of miscarriage and premature labour.[50] Any pregnancy achieved must be managed as high risk and needs expert obstetric care.

Sarcoma (osteosarcoma, Ewing's sarcoma and soft-tissue sarcomas)

Introduction

4.46 Sarcomas are uncommon tumours comprising 1–2% of malignancies. The bone sarcomas (osteosarcoma and Ewing's sarcoma) affect predominantly those in the adolescent years and early adulthood. Long-term survival will occur in 50–60% of patients with Ewing's sarcoma and 60–70% of patients with osteosarcoma. Soft-tissue sarcomas have their peak incidence in people in their 50s and 60s, but form a significant proportion of tumours affecting young adults. The cure rate for deep high-grade tumours is 50–60%. The treatment of these conditions is intensive and therefore has the potential for a significant adverse effect on fertility.

Management

4.47 Management depends upon accurate diagnosis and staging. Sarcoma therapy usually involves surgery with wide excision margins. Adjunctive therapy may include radical radiotherapy and chemotherapy. Reproductive health may be affected by chemotherapy and, in tumours of the pelvis, the consequences of local therapy (surgery or radiation).

Surgery

4.48 The impact of surgery on fertility depends on the site and any resultant damage to the genital tract.

Chemotherapy

4.49 *Osteosarcoma* is currently treated with cisplatin, doxorubicin and methotrexate as first-line therapy. Ifosfamide and etoposide may be used for poor responders or relapses. *Ewing's sarcoma* is currently treated with high-dose alkylating therapy. Drugs include vincristine, ifosfamide, etoposide, dactinomycin, cyclophosphamide and, in some patients, high-dose busulphan and melphalan. *Soft-tissue sarcomas* are a heterogeneous group of tumours that are frequently treated with ifosfamide- and anthracycline-based chemotherapy.[51]

4.50 All these combinations of therapies are likely to lead to significant reduction in male or female fertility. The extent is variable and will depend upon the combination of therapies. Consequently, all males should be offered sperm banking (sections 5.4–5.10) prior to being exposed to chemotherapy. Spermatogenesis may be maintained or return after therapy, although the use of significant cumulative doses of alkylating therapy (in Ewing's, soft-tissue sarcomas and relapsed/'poorly responding' osteosarcoma protocols) or high-dose therapy with busulphan and melphalan makes this less likely. Menstruation will be resumed in the majority of younger females, but early onset of menopause is likely. Where high-dose therapy or further treatment on relapse is used, ovarian failure is likely to be immediate and permanent. If time allows, females should be offered access to embryo/egg tissue storage (sections 5.19–5.26) However, Ewing's, osteosarcoma, and some soft-tissue sarcomas require urgent initiation of chemotherapy and these procedures may not be appropriate.

Radiotherapy

4.51 Radiotherapy to the pelvis and proximal thigh may adversely affect gamete production by direct or scattered irradiation. The doses required in these diseases are such that direct irradiation of the scrotum or penile bulb may produce endocrine or erectile dysfunction respectively, and of the uterus, inability to bear a pregnancy. Radiotherapy is routinely used as an adjuvant to radical surgery in deep and high-grade soft-tissue sarcoma. Most of these patients will not have had chemotherapy so sperm storage in males (sections 5.4–5.10) and oophoropexy or embryo/egg/ovarian storage (sections 5.19–5.26) in females should be considered where relevant. Radiation is indicated after radical surgery in Ewing's when margins are close or tumours inoperable and is, therefore, frequently used in pelvic primaries. All these patients will already have had chemotherapy and the males offered sperm storage. As recovery of ovarian function may be expected after this chemotherapy (except where high-dose therapy with stem cell support has been used), treatment will need to be individualised, but oophoropexy or embryo/egg/ovarian storage should be considered (sections 5.19–5.26) in females where radiotherapy is likely to obliterate the function of both ovaries.

Acute leukaemia

4.52   The acute leukaemias usually require urgent treatment with chemotherapy. In these circumstances sperm banking may still be possible (see sections 5.4–5.10). Egg, ovarian or gamete storage are usually inappropriate or practically impossible.

Acute lymphoblastic leukaemia

4.53   Acute lymphoblastic leukaemia (ALL) is a rare disease in adults, who account for only 20% of cases. Treatment requires multi-agent chemotherapy including daunorubicin, vincristine, steroids and asparaginase, with consolidation therapies with a number of drugs including cyclophosphamide, cytarabine, mercaptopurine, methotrexate and etoposide. Complete remissions are seen in 65–80% of patients, with long-term disease-free survival of approximately 35%. Treatment produces a significant impairment of reproductive function in men with early and usually complete recovery. Endocrine gonadal function remains unaffected. In women neither reproductive nor endocrine function is influenced in most cases.[52] In long-term survivors of childhood ALL, fertility is not commonly affected except in those exposed to high-dose irradiation.

Acute myeloid leukaemia

4.54   Acute myeloid leukaemia (AML) accounts for 80% of the acute leukaemias observed in adults, with an increasing incidence with age. Therapy of AML is more intensive than of ALL. To achieve complete remission, high doses of chemotherapy are delivered to induce profound hypoplasia. The basis of therapy is high-dose cytarabine in combination with an anthracycline. In addition, etoposide, thioguanine and more recently monoclonal antibodies are included in first or subsequent therapies. Usually four cycles of chemotherapy are delivered. For patients under 60 years of age, complete remission rates are achieved in around 80–85% of patients, with disease-free survival of around 40–50%. Infertility following this is reported in a small proportion of patients, with women more likely to be affected than men.

4.55   For men presenting with leukaemia, sperm storage should be routinely offered (sections 5.4–5.10). However, in women a biopsy of ovarian tissue will inevitably contain leukaemic cells and is not recommended, but could be considered when the disease is in remission.

Bone marrow transplantation

Autologous transplantation

4.56   Autologous transplantation is the treatment of choice for younger patients with relapsed forms of aggressive NHL, Hodgkin disease and myeloma. It is rarely used for other haematological malignancies or solid tumours. BEAM is the most commonly employed conditioning regimen in the UK. Total body irradiation (TBI) is rarely used in this setting. A few studies have looked at gonadal function post autograft. In the small numbers reported it appears that there is a high incidence of gonadal recovery in younger women who are menstruating at the time of the procedure, but azoospermia is almost always the rule in men. Post transplant the incidence of pregnancy is low (around 2%).[53] Most patients will have discussed issues relating to gamete storage and made appropriate arrangements at an earlier stage in their disease management.

Allogeneic transplantation

4.57   Allogeneic transplantation, using either a sibling or unrelated volunteer donor, is commonly employed in acute leukaemias at relapse or in high-risk patients as part of initial therapy. It is the recognised curative treatment for chronic myeloid leukaemia and is increasingly being employed in the lymphoproliferative disorders including indolent lymphomas and chronic lymphatic leukaemia, particularly as safer ways of delivering the transplant are being developed. Conditioning regimens commonly involve TBI or myeloablative doses of cyclophosphamide and busulphan. Approximately 40–60% of patients receiving a transplant survive five years afterwards and the vast majority of these will be long-term survivors.

4.58   Most patients receiving TBI conditioning have gonadal failure. In women this causes durable ovarian damage with hypergonadotrophic ovarian failure and lasting infertility. Gonadal function can recover in 10–14% of women, but pregnancies are very unusual. In men, recovery of gonadal function has been reported in less than 20% of patients.[54] However, long-term follow-up has shown evidence of recovering spermatogenesis in one series (median 9 years) where approximately 50% of patients demonstrated recovery.[55] However, fathering a child is a rare event for such patients.

4.59   The combination of busulphan and cyclophosphamide produces a similarly high incidence of gonadal failure. In women, recovery of gonadal function is rare and no pregnancies have been reported following this treatment for patients with leukaemia. In men, return of gonadal function occurs in a similar percentage to post-TBI and a few patients have fathered children naturally. In addition to the specific toxic effects of the conditioning therapies used for allogeneic bone marrow transplant, patients do suffer long-term effects of the transplant, specifically graft versus host disease, which will have an additional impact on sexual function and hence fertility.

4.60   Reduced intensity allogeneic transplantation is increasingly being used. This employs no ablative conditioning, using fludarabine in combination with melphalan, busulphan and cyclophosphamide or BEAM often in combination with the antibody alemtuzumab. This is currently predominantly used in more elderly patients; however, there is evidence that the efficacy of this approach is similar to that seen with conventionally conditioned allografting. It is likely, therefore, that this will be employed in younger patients in the future with a significantly lower risk of gonadal damage.

5 Recommended procedures before commencing chemotherapy/radiotherapy likely to affect fertility

5.1 The possible future effects of chemotherapy or radiotherapy on fertility should be discussed with all patients with reproductive potential. It should be recognised that the prospect of infertility can be psychologically and socially damaging for both men and women, but that such an outcome can, to some extent, be mitigated by gamete and embryo storage. Discussions of these issues may be difficult in a number of circumstances, particularly in the case of adolescent patients or patients with incurable cancer. These discussions should take place in private, should involve appropriate family members or other individuals and, where possible, should be conducted by experienced, preferably trained, staff. Specialist psychological support and counselling should be available. Additional problems may arise in patients for whom English is not their first language.

5.2 Effective contraceptive precautions should be recommended in all males and females once treatment is commenced and for at least one year after it is completed.

5.3 This section describes a number of well validated and widely used approaches to preserve fertility, eg sperm storage or embryo storage, and some approaches that are less widely available (testicular sperm retrieval) or currently in development (egg storage, ovarian strip storage). There is currently no national funding policy for any of these techniques. Although sperm banking is widely available (though not necessarily funded), provision of the other techniques is patchy or absent. An agreed national policy and equity of access are highly desirable.

Males

Sperm storage

5.4 The likely effects of treatment with chemotherapy or radiotherapy on fertility should be discussed with all male patients. All postpubertal males who may develop gonadal dysfunction, should, whenever relevant, be offered sperm banking.

5.5 Proxy consent cannot be given for the collection and storage of sperm. For this reason, individuals who are under the age of legal consent for medical intervention (18 years in England, Wales and Northern Ireland, 16 years in Scotland) must be involved in these discussions as they alone can provide legal consent. Adolescent patients have the same rights to privacy as adults and may prefer not to discuss, for example, sperm banking, with their parents present. Capacity to provide written consent will need to be determined by the health professionals caring for the individual. Assessment should be based on *Gillick* criteria (Gillick v West Norfolk and Wisbech Area Health Authority 1985). Involvement of a paediatric psychologist, specialist paediatric nurse or fertility specialist may be useful in cases where the clinical team are uncertain as to the patient's competence/capacity to provide this.

5.6   A sperm storage facility together with counselling resources should be available to all cancer centres and units. In the past, arbitrary limits on sperm concentrations suitable for freezing were set, but following advances in IVF and in particular ICSI, any number of sperm (whatever the quality) should be considered for storage.

5.7   In general it is recommended that at least two semen samples are collected over a period of one week and stored before treatment for cancer. Males should be sexually abstinent where possible for at least two days before each collection. The Human Fertility and Embryology Authority (HFEA) recommends that semen samples be produced on site wherever possible. In exceptional circumstances they can be produced at home, if delivered to the laboratory within 30–45 minutes of production.

5.8   In patients with advanced cancer, or those where there is an urgent need to start treatment, it may only be possible to store one sample before commencing treatment. In some situations, the individual may be too unwell to provide a semen sample prior to exposure to cytotoxic therapy. If it is decided to attempt sperm storage following exposure to any systemic cytotoxic therapy, this exposure must be clearly recorded by the sperm bank. The DNA damaging effects of cytotoxic therapy cannot currently be established and the sample may not be appropriate for subsequent use. Individuals should be warned of this before providing a sample for storage. Future developments may possibly enable the integrity of sperm DNA to be examined and therefore provide more information with respect to this.

5.9   Prior to sperm banking all patients must be tested serologically for evidence of HIV, hepatitis B and C and syphilis. In urgent cases sperm banking can take place in a separate vessel while these results are obtained.

5.10   Sperm banking is usually available on the NHS. However, this is not always the case and so services may only be available in the private sector.

Testicular sperm retrieval

5.11   Patients found to be azoospermic can, in some cases, have limited sperm production within the testis. Serum FSH levels provide some indication as to the likely success of testicular sperm retrieval (TSR), but even when levels are elevated sperm can, on occasion, be obtained for ICSI. Sperm can be extracted either by aspiration of the testis under local anaesthetic or by an open surgical approach with microdissection of the seminiferous tubules. TSR has been used successfully both before chemotherapy and after treatment.[45] Currently TSR is not widely funded by the NHS.

Legal aspects

5.12   Sperm can only be stored and used in a centre licensed by the HFEA (**www.hfea.gov.uk**). All patients need to complete HFEA consent forms covering the storage and use of the stored samples and such consent can only be obtained by a member of staff named on the sperm bank licence. All patients banking sperm whose fertility is likely to be impaired as a result of chemotherapy/radiotherapy need to complete and sign HFEA form MS, which provides consent for sperm storage. This form does not cover consent for use of the samples; before the stored sperm can be used in treatment services, consent for use must be obtained (HFEA form MT). This form giving consent for use (MT) also details the generation of embryos *in vitro* and the fate of these embryos if the man dies or is unable because of incapacity to vary the terms of consent or revoke it. The patient may vary their consent at any time, but must inform the centre storing the samples in writing.

5.13   Current legislation permits the storage of sperm for up to 10 years for any patient regardless of age. This period can be extended for individuals whose fertility has been or is likely to be impaired by treatment for cancer and who are less than 45 years old when the gametes are produced. The continued storage of sperm is not permitted beyond the patient's 55th birthday.

5.14   In order for a woman to use her deceased partner's sperm for treatment, the man must have given consent to the posthumous use of his sperm for that purpose/treatment (form MT). In the event of the sperm being used after the man is dead, the man is not treated as the father of the child that results from the use of the sperm, except for the purpose of being recorded as the father of the child on the register of births. In order to be recorded on a birth certificate as the father, section 6 of the MT form must be completed.

5.15   It is an HFEA requirement that all males banking sperm should be offered independent counselling by a suitably qualified individual and receive oral and written explanation about the medical, scientific, legal and psychosocial implications of their decision (with leaflets in an appropriate language level for adolescents). Discussion with a patient should include a description of the process of freezing, storing the samples and the patient's ability to change their consent. It should be made clear that there is no guarantee of intact sperm function after thawing and that the patient's illness itself may affect sperm quality. It is, however, possible to store sperm for many years without the quality being compromised. The patient should be advised, where appropriate, that the recovery of fertility is possible following treatment and that they can be offered further counselling at a later stage if required. Patients should also receive information about options available in the event of death or mental incapacity and the consent required to fulfil these wishes. They should also receive specific information appropriate to minors.

5.16   The comments above apply equally to women storing eggs. There are complex psychological issues for the recipient of donated eggs or sperm.

5.17   At the counselling session the appropriate HFEA factsheet should be provided and a copy of the completed forms (HFEA MS, MT) given to the patient.

5.18   In order to maintain accurate records the oncologist should provide full medical details about the patient as well as full details of where the details of the sperm count should be sent. It is important also for the semen bank to maintain accurate up-to-date records of the status of the patient as well as to establish whether the sperm should be destroyed should the patient die. The centre will need to keep in contact with the patient, particularly towards the end of the statutory 10-year period, to see whether samples should be destroyed or whether storage for a further period of years is necessary.

Females

5.19   The ovary is more resistant to the effects of chemotherapy and irradiation than the testis. Preservation of fertility by egg storage would be a useful technique prior to treatment, but no non-invasive method of fertility preservation analogous to sperm cryopreservation is currently available.[56,57]

Embryo storage

5.20   The legal requirements that apply to sperm storage also apply to egg storage and embryo storage. It is a legal requirement that non-medical counselling should be available to all patients.

5.21   The best validated technique is egg harvesting and fertilisation with sperm of a partner or donor: the resulting embryos can be cryopreserved long-term with good results following embryo transfer. There are, however, a number of drawbacks to this approach. The procedure involves hormonal administration to induce multiple follicular development (superovulation), and oocyte recovery which is generally performed trans-vaginally under local anaesthetic. These manipulations take a minimum of 2–4 weeks (plus additional time for referral) and this may be an unacceptable delay for many patients. Sperm are also required, which may not be available, or may raise ethical or legal issues regarding involvement and level of commitment of the male partner. There are concerns about the very high oestradiol levels attained during superovulation as this may accelerate growth, for example of oestrogen receptor positive breast cancer. Research studies suggest that the use of FSH with tamoxifen or letrozole may result in lower oestrogen levels with satisfactory egg harvests.[58] NHS funding may be available for embryo storage.

Egg or ovarian tissue storage

5.22   In most cases, because of timing considerations or absence of a partner, production of embryos will not be realistic and egg or ovarian storage may be considered. It should be emphasised that neither of these techniques is available on a routine basis in the NHS and both should be regarded as at an early stage of use/research.

Egg storage

5.23   Oocytes (eggs) are much more vulnerable to damage from cryopreservation than sperm, reflecting their large size and inherent chromosome instability. Ongoing technical developments have led to increased success rates, but this procedure is not widely available. Oocytes are obtained from mature follicles after induction of superovulation using FSH as with IVF. Obtaining oocytes by this route takes 2–4 weeks, which may be a source of concern in many oncology patients. In addition, success rates are lower than with embryo cryopreservation and the safety of the child conceived cannot be assured particularly in the light of evidence of an increased incidence of imprinting defects associated with assisted conception (though not with gamete storage). On average 10 oocytes may be retrieved following stimulation, but with live birth rates of less than 5% per oocyte. These poor results are reflected in total live delivery worldwide of little more than a hundred infants after use of this technique.[2] Immature oocytes obtained with reduced or no stimulation are now being used for fertility treatment in some centres and successful cryopreservation has been reported. This potentially offers a considerable time-saving and addresses concerns regarding possible effects of high oestradial levels in cancer patients.

Ovarian tissue storage

5.24   This is at a research stage and some way from entering standard clinical practice.[59] Ovarian tissue may be obtained at laparoscopy and cryopreserved. Potential advantages of this compared to embryo cryopreservation are that it does not require hormone treatment so may be quicker and applicable to younger/prepubertal girls, and a male partner is not required. Following successful completion of cancer therapy ovarian tissue may be re-implanted in the pelvis or heterotopically, eg subcutaneously, in the anterior abdominal wall. A thorough pathological assessment of the tissue must be performed to exclude the presence of metastatic disease. Most follicles are lost due to ischaemia during re-vascularisation. The limited data available indicate that when the transplant has been successful, follicular activity may be detected after several months. Successful live births have been reported after both spontaneous conception and IVF.[59]

5.25   Storage of ovarian tissue is not covered by the HFEA as it does not contain mature gametes but it is covered by the Human Tissue Authority (**www.hta.gov.uk**). Storage of such tissue is subject to tissue banking regulations and its availability is therefore very restricted. Several professional bodies have produced guidelines relevant to ovarian tissue cryopreservation[56,57] emphasising that this promising approach is some way from being sufficiently established to be appropriate to offer as part of a clinical service, but should be developed within the context of clinical trials with defined inclusion and exclusion criteria. It is currently very unclear which patients are the most appropriate candidates for this option and what the most appropriate surgical techniques are.

5.26   There is a need for an organised and research-based approach to egg and ovarian strip storage. The success of these techniques is developmental and likely to improve. Widespread access to a centrally funded, evidence-based, finite number of centres would be highly advantageous for this patient group.

6 Management of post-treatment infertility

Introduction

6.1   For many patients, post-treatment fertility is not a source of concern. Most patients with cancer are beyond the childbearing years, or will have completed their family.

6.2   Patients wishing to have children should be carefully advised both before and after treatment has been completed. Important issues to be discussed include the response to treatment, likely prognosis and the effects of the given therapy on fertility.

6.3   There is currently no evidence that cancer treatments increase the incidence of birth defects in children conceived after treatment has been completed. It is generally recommended, however, that male or female patients delay starting a family for a minimum of one year after cancer treatment, mainly because of concern about relapse, but also because of the possible mutagenic effects of treatment on the gametes.

6.4   In many women menstrual function and fertility will be little affected by anti-cancer treatments. Where gonadal irradiation or gonadotoxic systemic chemotherapy have been given, menstrual dysfunction and a significant reduction in reproductive lifespan with a premature menopause can occur. Those who develop irregular and troublesome menstruation should be assessed in the normal manner, which may require referral to the gynaecology clinic. This may require imaging of the uterine cavity and endometrial biopsy. Some forms of menstrual irregularity may respond well to exogenous hormone regimens. The use of oestrogen would be contraindicated in a patient with a history of breast cancer.

6.5   Female patients receiving gonadotoxic treatments but who wish to have children and in whom menstruation returns should be advised to consider starting a family within a reasonably short time span (although not under one year from treatment, see above) because of the risk of premature menopause. Patients should be aware that the normal decline in fertility that begins in women in their mid-thirties is likely to be accelerated following chemotherapy.

6.6   Male patients are more often adversely affected than women by gonadal radiotherapy or chemotherapy. Recovery of sperm count, where this occurs, may take years. Androgen production is usually much less affected.

Supportive techniques available to sub-fertile/infertile couples after cancer treatments

Artificial insemination by husband's/partner's cryopreserved semen

6.7   Artificial insemination using husband's/partner's (AIH) cryopreserved semen is a widely available technique generally funded by the NHS. Where adequate quantities of sperm have been banked, aliquots of this are injected into the cervix or uterus at the time of ovulation. Many clinics stimulate ovulation with drugs to induce more than one follicle per cycle. Although AIH is used, there is an increasing tendency to use IVF and ICSI to treat couples who have stored sperm.

6.8   In the event of the death of the patient whose sperm is banked, it is important to realise that subsequent re-insemination of the wife/partner can only take place if the man has provided explicit written consent to use. There is no obligation on the HFEA-licensed centre to perform the treatment. Registered clinics will be prepared to pass samples on to another clinic that has agreed to perform such insemination. Where a woman is treated with her dead husband's or partner's sperm he will not be treated as the legal father (see section 5.14).

Donor insemination

6.9   Donor insemination is widely available in HFEA-licensed centres and may be considered for women whose husband/partner has been sterilised by treatment and where cryopreserved sperm are unavailable. Sperm is provided by donors (who are registered with the HFEA). Donors are usually matched for racial and physical characteristics. Sperm is inseminated into the cervix or into the uterus. Similarly, egg or embryo donation may be available to women sterilised by cancer treatment.

6.10   As a result of new legislation, from 2006 all sperm donors will be identifiable (except when using gametes to create genetically related siblings for existing children). The donor has no legal obligation to the resulting child but the child has the right to obtain identifiable information about the donor (including name and contact details) once s/he is 18 years old. There has recently been a considerable diminution in the availability of donor sperm. There are complex psychological and ethical issues relating to the creation of families by donation and an offer of counselling is a requirement of the Human Fertilisation and Embryology Act 1990.

IVF/ICSI

6.11   Where only small quantities of cryopreserved sperm are available (as will commonly be the case), IVF/ICSI may be considered. ICSI involves injection of a single sperm into each oocyte. Pregnancy results are generally favourable (28% for women under 35 years of age). The most important risks to these children are associated with multiple pregnancy, especially from pre-term delivery. Assessment of singleton ICSI and IVF children at five years of age has been generally reassuring. However, ICSI children may have a slightly increased risk of congenital malformations (particularly in the male) and both ICSI and IVF children are more likely to need healthcare resources than naturally conceived children.[60,61]

Egg donation

6.12   In women whose ovarian reserve has been severely depleted, eg by chemotherapy, and who have elevated FSH concentrations, superovulation for IVF is generally unsuccessful.

6.13   For these women who are peri- or postmenopausal egg donation is required. Chemotherapy has no effect on the uterus, which is able to support implantation and successful pregnancy once appropriate exogenous hormones have been administered to prepare the endometrium. This treatment should be maintained for at least the first seven weeks of pregnancy, after which the placenta will take over. In contrast, radiotherapy of the uterus increases the risk of miscarriage and premature delivery.

Role of the HFEA

6.14   The HFEA is the national licensing authority for all clinics that store human gametes or provide IVF/ICSI treatment or donor insemination. The HFEA website (**www.hfea.gov.uk**) contains a wealth of information with clinical leaflets on sperm storage, treatment options, a list of all HFEA clinics and a guide to infertility.

7 Alternative means of family increase

Surrogacy

7.1   Surrogacy is where another woman carries a baby for an infertile couple. It is legal in the UK, but infrequently used.

7.2   Surrogacy is described as traditional (also known as 'straight') when the surrogate mother provides the egg (and is therefore the genetic mother of the child) and sperm is donated by the female patient's partner. In full surrogacy (also known as 'gestational' or 'host') the surrogate mother carries an embryo from the commissioning couple. Occasionally the embryo may be derived from egg or sperm donation.

7.3   The surrogate mother is the legal mother of the child at birth (and her husband, if she has one, is the legal father). For the commissioning parents to acquire legal parenthood status, the surrogate mother must have agreed to the granting of a Parental Order between six weeks and six months after the birth of the child, enabling the commissioning couple to have full legal rights in relationship to the child. It is legally permissible for 'reasonable expenses' of the surrogate mother to be met by the commissioning parents, but any payments to either the surrogate mother or a third party are not.

Adoption

7.4   In the UK very few babies are available for adoption. Patients cured of cancer are not excluded from consideration by adoption agencies, but careful consideration will be given to the needs of the child and waiting lists are likely to be long. Parents considering adoption of older children or children with special needs may be considered more readily.

International adoption

7.5   International adoption is a possibility but there may be considerable difficulties. It can be a complex and expensive process although some countries have reciprocal arrangements with the UK. Applications to adopt a child must be approved by the Home Office and local adoption agencies, usually social services.

8 Hormone replacement following gonadal damage

Diagnosis and management of premature menopause

8.1   Premature ovarian failure or menopause is the development of amenorrhoea, with concomitant sex hormone deficiency and elevated serum gonadotrophin levels, at the age of 40 years or younger. This occurs naturally in about 1% of women and can be spontaneous or induced by chemotherapy, radiation therapy or oophorectomy. A premature menopause, from all causes, is associated with an earlier onset of osteoporosis and coronary heart disease. HRT should therefore be offered to these women. In a recent Royal College of Obstetricians and Gynaecologists (RCOG) Study Group consensus statement on menopause and hormone replacement,[62] it was concluded that hormone replacement should be used in younger women (under 40 years) who had experienced a premature menopause unless contraindicated (see section 4.12 for comments about breast cancer) and for treating menopausal symptoms and preventing osteoporosis until the age of normal menopause, when therapy should be reviewed. Natural menopause is defined retrospectively as the last menstrual period before the absence of menses for 12 consecutive months, without obvious cause (eg pregnancy), and it usually occurs at about 50 years of age.

8.2   HRT following development of a treatment-induced menopause is currently not exempt from prescription charges. It is recommended that this policy be brought into line with other long-term replacement therapies by the introduction of such an exemption.

8.3   The most appropriate means of assessing hormonal status is by measuring FSH and oestradiol concentrations. If amenorrhoea persists for more than six months with elevated FSH (>30 U/L) and low oestradiol (<100 pmol/L) concentrations, the patient is menopausal and HRT with an oestrogen only (if no uterus) or oestrogen plus progestogen regimen should be considered, assuming no contraindication to administration of exogenous oestrogen. During the perimenopausal transition, which may last for several years in these women, fluctuating FSH and oestradiol concentrations will be frequently recorded and occasional ovulatory cycles may occur. If oestradiol concentrations are persistently over 150 pmol/L then oestradiol supplementation is not required for prevention of osteoporosis. HRT is not contraceptive. If there is any possibility of spontaneous return of cyclical ovarian activity, with ovulatory cycles and therefore a potential need for contraception, then HRT in the form of a combined oral contraceptive preparation should be used (with assessment of contraindications as per usual practice).

8.4   The diagnosis of premature ovarian failure may be unclear in women taking exogenous sex steroids (contraceptive pill, HRT, oral or systemic progestogens). Under these circumstances measurement of serum gonadotrophins may be difficult to interpret. This can be made more certain by timing the blood sample to be at the end of a pill-free week or ideally 2–3 weeks following discontinuation of exogenous sex steroids.

8.5   It should be noted that the levonorgestrel-releasing intrauterine system (LNG-IUS; Mirena® system) does not inhibit ovulation and suppress gonadotrophins. The circulating levels of progestogen (LNG) with this intrauterine hormone delivery system are extremely low and therefore progestogenic side effects are minimal. The exception is unscheduled breakthrough bleeding as experienced by about a fifth of all women using exogenous progestogen preparations. There is no specific intervention for this nuisance side effect and good counselling prior to use of the LNG-IUS, and indeed all progestogen-only prescriptions, is most important. Many women will see an improvement in breakthrough bleeding within six months of commencement of intrauterine LNG delivery. The LNG-IUS is an excellent contraceptive with the added health benefit of reduced menstrual blood loss. Hence its contemporary widespread use as a management option for heavy menstrual bleeding and as the progestogen component of HRT when oestrogen replacement is either oral or via a transdermal delivery route.

▶   There are still many gaps in our knowledge about the optimal management of women with premature ovarian failure. Outstanding questions include:

–   What form and dose of hormone replacement is most appropriate – combination oral contraception, continuous menopausal hormone replacement or sequential therapy?

–   What is the optimal length of time that hormone replacement should be administered?

Long-term follow-up of women with premature ovarian failure should be considered and studies carried out to answer some of the questions.

8.6   A variety of hormone replacement therapies are available. In general, combined (oestrogen and progestogen) preparations are indicated in women with an intact uterus, and oestrogen-only preparations in women following hysterectomy. Oral preparations, patches and implants (lasting 3–6 months) are available. Many preparations allow for a period of withdrawal bleeding at monthly intervals – other preparations allow bleeding once every three months and newer 'no bleed' preparations are available. Continuous combined preparations are often associated with a complaint of unscheduled breakthrough bleeding, albeit often minimal in nature, but still perceived as a nuisance factor by the patient.

Testosterone replacement therapy in male cancer survivors

8.7   Only a small minority of male patients will become hypogonadal as a result of cancer treatment; patients with testicular cancer or those with hypothalamic/pituitary damage are most at risk. The clinical manifestations of hypogonadism in the male are infertility and the consequences of testosterone deficiency (Table 1). Hypogonadism can be secondary to gonadotrophin deficiency due to pituitary/hypothalamic disease and its treatment, or due to primary testicular failure in which serum gonadotrophins levels are elevated. Spermatogenesis is more sensitive to testicular damage than testosterone synthesis by Leydig cells and if testosterone deficiency occurs it will always be preceded by infertility. There is increasing appreciation of the consequences of partial androgen deficiency and the benefits of treatment. All features of testosterone deficiency should be reversible with appropriate testosterone replacement therapy.[63,64]

Table I Clinical manifestations of hypogonadism in the male.	
Pubertal	**Postpubertal**
Delayed puberty	Slowing of hair growth; hair recession and balding halted or slowed
Small phallus	
Scant pubic/axillary hair	Progressive decrease in muscle mass
Delayed epiphyseal closure: disproportionately long limbs	Erectile dysfunction
	Loss of energy
Reduced male musculature	Loss of libido
Gynaecomastia	Reduction in concentration
High-pitched voice	Changes in mood
	Reduction in bone mineral density
	Reduction in lean body mass
	Increase in visceral fat

Investigation of suspect testosterone deficiency

8.8   The interpretation of serum testosterone levels is complicated as circulating testosterone has a circadian rhythm with peak levels being seen in the early morning, and 99% is bound to sex hormone binding globulin (SHBG), albumin and other plasma proteins with only the 1% that is free being biologically active. Therefore factors that alter SHBG will alter total but not bioactive testosterone. SHBG levels fall with obesity, glucocorticoid therapy, hyperinsulinaemia and hypothyroidism and are elevated by oestrogens and hyperthyroidism. Free testosterone measurement is not routinely available and therefore at diagnosis all patients should have testosterone plus SHBG measured between 07.00 and 11.00 hours. Gonadotrophin measurement is necessary to distinguish between primary and secondary hypogonadism, and results should always be interpreted in conjunction with symptoms. If the serum testosterone level is within the reference range but the serum LH level is elevated, patients should be re-tested every 3–6 months and testosterone replacement started if there is a declining trend. Assessment of bone density should be considered in all hypogonadal males as repeat assessment may be of value in monitoring the response to treatment.

Forms of androgen replacement therapy

8.9   The goal of testosterone replacement therapy is to imitate normal physiology. This treatment is lifelong. Comparable long-term replacement therapies (eg thyroxine) are centrally funded, but testosterone is not. We strongly recommend that prescriptions of this drug should be exempted from standard charges, bringing it into line with other, comparable, drugs.

8.10   Androgens are metabolised very rapidly by the liver and are therefore ineffective when given orally; for this reason they are delivered either transdermally or parentally. For many years intramuscular testosterone esters have been the most widely used form of replacement therapy, but they have the inherent disadvantage of inappropriately high post-injection peak levels and sub-therapeutic nadir values prior to the following injection. The testosterone esters can result in injection site tenderness.

8.11   Implants, normally administered every six months, have been available for a long time and suit some patients' lifestyles, but require insertion by a specialist nurse and judging the dosing interval can be difficult. More recently a three-monthly intramuscular depot testosterone preparation has become available.

8.12   Transdermal testosterone preparations are the most popular form of replacement therapy as they are convenient and provide consistent plasma testosterone concentrations. A testosterone patch was the first of these newer generation preparations, but its acceptability has been limited by local skin reactions, adhesion problems and the stigma associated with patch wearing. Testosterone gels applied once daily are very popular; a buccal tablet, that is changed twice daily, is an alternative and provides similarly consistent serum testosterone levels.[64]

How often to test for testosterone deficiency

8.13   All postpubertal patients at risk of primary testicular failure should be offered pre-treatment cryopreservation of sperm. At the same time, baseline serum testosterone should be measured as that may provide evidence of pre-existing gonadal failure for unrelated reasons and a baseline value for subsequent comparison. Chemotherapy and testicular irradiation can induce rapid failure in spermatogenesis, but testosterone deficiency develops more slowly. Irradiation encompassing the pituitary, over the course of years, will result in hypopituitarism, with gonadotrophin deficiency being one of the first manifestations; serum testosterone should be measured on an annual basis.

Judging the effectiveness of replacement therapy

8.14   Monitoring of symptoms, particularly tiredness, libido and erectile function including early morning erections, is fundamental to monitoring therapy. Serum testosterone measurement is of value with the transdermal preparations as levels should be constant. With the parenteral preparations, serum testosterone levels will fluctuate in relationship to the interval since the last dose and their main value is in judging the timing of the next dose.

Risks of testosterone therapy

8.15   Patients on testosterone therapy should be on lifelong annual review to ensure the safety and efficacy of treatment, and to ensure that patients are aware of the increasing variety of preparations available.

8.16   The effect of testosterone treatment on the risk of prostate cancer is a subject of intense study. Hypogonadal men are at less risk of benign prostatic hyperplasia and carcinoma. There is no evidence that physiological testosterone replacement therapy increases the risk beyond that in the background population. The risk of prostate disease increases with age and therefore great caution is required in the older male. Prostate-specific antigen (PSA) should be measured annually and will frequently rise with initiation of testosterone therapy, but should remain within the reference range. In men over 45 years of age, digital rectal examination should be performed at baseline while PSA should be monitored at 3, 6 and 12 months and then annually. Testosterone therapy should be discontinued in the presence of malignant prostate disease.[65]

8.17   Testosterone stimulates haemopoiesis, and polycythaemia is a risk of over-treatment so it is recommended that patients should have annual haemoglobin measurement.

9 Cancer and pregnancy

9.1   Pregnancy is occasionally complicated by a diagnosis of cancer, with breast cancer and lymphoma the two most common malignancies encountered. Additionally, around 1 in 1,000 pregnancies are complicated by gestational trophoblastic disease (GTD), an abnormal proliferation of trophoblastic tissue that usually presents as a miscarriage. Rarely GTD and a viable fetus can coexist, or the diagnosis may be made postpartum.

9.2   Treatment of cancer during pregnancy requires careful consideration of the risk of the disease and gestational age of the fetus by a multidisciplinary care team, in conjunction with the patient's preferences. In breast cancer, surgical management is usually sufficient initial management and chemotherapy can be postponed until after delivery. However, in lymphoma and occasional inoperable or metastatic breast cancers, it may be necessary to administer chemotherapy during pregnancy.

9.3   Chemotherapy should be deferred beyond the first trimester as it has a high risk of miscarriage or severe fetal abnormality.[66] Administration of cyclophosphamide during the second trimester has also been reported to result in fetal demise, but most infants exposed *in utero* to combination chemotherapy seem to suffer no major long-term detrimental consequences.[67] Anthracyclines, taxanes, vinca alkaloids and trastuzumab have all been used in the later stages of pregnancy without obvious immediate untoward effects on the fetus. However, the impact of fetal exposure to chemotherapy on the rate of malignancy, cardiac function and subsequent fertility are poorly defined.

9.4   It is likely that chemotherapy regimens known to have detrimental effects on the prepubertal testis and ovary would also have effects *in utero*, but both of these would be difficult to detect without follow-up into adulthood, which is not available. Potentially in women, reproductive lifespan might be affected as the primordial follicle pool is formed during the second trimester of pregnancy and in men spermatogenesis might be reduced.

10 Pregnancy and offspring after cancer treatment

10.1   Following cancer therapy, there are concerns regarding the potential for increased risks in pregnancy to the mother and her unborn progeny. However, there does not appear to be an excess risk of death in survivors of childhood cancer during subsequent pregnancies.

10.2   It is recommended that the history of the malignant disease, and its treatment, should be flagged up with the obstetric team supervising the care of the cancer survivor. Management by a 'high-risk' obstetric service should be considered.

10.3   The risks of cancer treatments and management of those areas of risk in pregnancy and in offspring are summarised in Tables 2a and 2b.

Table 2a Potential risks to pregnancy after cancer treatment.			
Area of potential adverse outcome	**Cause/therapeutic exposure**	**Potential risk**	**Screening/ management**
Breast and lactation	*Radiation* • chest wall • upper abdominal/flank • whole lung	Reduced lactation[68] Breast hypoplasia (if radiation prior to completion of breast development)	Advise women antenatally of potential difficulties
Cardiac function	*Chemotherapy* • anthracyclines *Radiation* • mediastinal • chest • scatter from high abdominal	Cardiac decompensation, especially during first and third trimesters and peripartum[69–71]	Echocardiogram and resting ECG when pregnancy is detected and at beginning of third trimester, and as clinically indicated Monitoring by high-risk obstetric service and cardiologists
Musculoskeletal	*Radiation* • abdominal in childhood	Truncal shortening and muscular hypoplasia Potential difficulties in labour	Monitoring by high-risk obstetric service
Pulmonary function	*Chemotherapy* • bleomycin • busulphan • BCNU • CCNU	Restrictive lung defect	Pulmonary function tests pre-conception (if possible)

continued

Table 2a Potential risks to pregnancy after cancer treatment. – continued

Area of potential adverse outcome	Cause/therapeutic exposure	Potential risk	Screening/ management
Pulmonary function	*Radiation* • whole lung • mediastinal • mantle • total body • craniospinal	Pulmonary fibrosis	Discussion with anaesthetists if patient had bleomycin exposure. This can lead to acute respiratory decompensation with subsequent exposure to high oxygen concentration.
Renal function	*Nephrotoxic chemotherapy* *Radiation* • pelvic • flank • abdominal	Renal insufficiency[72]	Monitoring renal function
Uterine function	*Radiation* • pelvic • total body irradiation • scatter from abdominal	Reduced vascularity and poor uterine elasticity resulting in: • increased risk of spontaneous miscarriage • *in utero* growth retardation • premature labour • low birth weight[54,73]	Early referral to a high-risk obstetric service

BCNU = bis-chloroethyl-nitrosourea (carmustine); CCNU = chloroethyl-cyclohexyl-nitrosourea (lomutine); ECG = electrocardiogram.

Table 2b Potential risks to offspring conceived after treatment.

Potential adverse outcome	Cause/therapeutic exposure	Potential risk	Screening/ management
Adverse health outcomes in offspring	*Chemotherapy*	*Chemotherapy* No increased risk of cancer or congenital abnormalities in offspring of female survivors 5 years or more from completion of therapy[74,75]	
	Radiation • pelvis • abdominal radiation (if scatter)	• *In utero* growth retardation • Fetus small for gestational age[76,77]	

continued

Table 2b Potential risks to offspring conceived after treatment. – *continued*

Potential adverse outcome	Cause/therapeutic exposure	Potential risk	Screening/ management
Malignancy	*Genetic predisposition syndromes*	There appears to be no increased risk of cancer in offspring of survivors of cancer, unless there is evidence of a genetic predisposition[78]	Appropriate cancer genetics counselling. Screening of offspring if a predisposition syndrome exists
Teratogenicity	*Cytotoxic drugs or radiation during first trimester* Exposure after first trimester may affect growth and development[6]	Significant developmental abnormalities	Early referral and joint management between oncology and feto-maternal medicine teams

11 Potential future directions for preservation of fertility

11.1 In the nine years since our last report,[4] there have been important developments in potential fertility-preserving therapies for patients exposed to sterilising cancer treatment. Much of this progress has related to work in animals, and data from human material have been limited. However, our knowledge of germ cell biology (development and function) is rapidly expanding, particularly in the light of the breathtaking progress in adult and embryonic stem cell research. This knowledge is likely to result in rapid progress in the next five years. The following sections describe areas where progress is being made and we will need to re-evaluate our practices with increasing frequency.

Male

11.2 The testis contains a small population of spermatogonial stem cells, which can, in animal species, be isolated, cryopreserved and reintroduced into the sterilised testis resulting in restoration of spermatogenesis.[79] Alternatively, testicular cell suspensions can re-form spermatogenic tubules following xenografting, with the production of functional sperm.[80] Application of these techniques to the human is potentially relevant to prepubertal boys. However, in adults it may be appropriate where storage of ejaculated or testicular sperm is not possible, and offers the possibility of restoration of fertility not limited by a finite number of sperm cryopreserved before treatment.

Female

Cryopreservation of human eggs (oocytes)

11.3 Mature human oocyte cryopreservation has met with limited success.[81] Overall there is a live birth rate per oocyte thawed of approximately 2%. However, this is an area of intense research with some research groups reporting relatively higher success rates.[82] Improved and shared practice along with inevitable advances encompassing, for example, better cryopreservation regimes (eg vitrification) and freezing of immature oocytes, suggests that oocyte cryopreservation is likely to become a realistic option for preservation of fertility within the next five years. This is likely to be applicable to prepubertal girls as well as adult women.

In vitro maturation

11.4 Developments in *in vitro* maturation (IVM) methods for human oocytes prior to IVF/ICSI have greatly improved success rates.[83] This allows the recovery of immature oocytes without the need for gonadotrophin stimulation, thus allowing more flexibility and less time-consuming hormonal manipulations for the recovery of potentially viable oocytes for assisted conception. Although data are limited, the children born from these procedures appear normal.[84] In combination with the inevitable further improvements in oocyte culture conditions this will make the recovery of immature eggs followed by IVM a realistic option for patients who need to start chemotherapy without delay.

Ovarian tissue storage and autologous transplantation

11.5 Live births have now been reported following ovarian tissue cryopreservation and autotransplantation.[59] In both cases, ovarian tissue was returned to the pelvis. Reimplantation to other sites, including subcutaneously in the forearm and in the abdominal wall, have also resulted in follicular development, and successful embryo development after aspiration and ICSI.[85] It appears that the dynamics of follicular development are altered in those environments, but further advances will undoubtedly result in successful pregnancy. Improvements in other methods of oocyte preservation discussed above may make this approach most suited to the prepubertal girl. New molecular markers may give greater accuracy in detecting tissue contamination by malignant cells. In addition to developments in these technologies, much more accurate information needs to be obtained regarding the effects of cancer therapies on the ovary, to enable appropriate patient selection.

11.6 Live births from oocytes grown *in vitro* and subsequently matured have been reported in mice,[86] but despite improvements the techniques remain experimental and are not yet robust and clearly defined. In humans there is a marked paucity of knowledge on the conditions necessary for *in vitro* growth and although rapid progress is likely in animals, for example in developing new culture systems,[87] it is unlikely that robust procedures for the *in vitro* growth of human oocytes will be available in the next five years.

Development of mature functional gametes from adult or embryonic stem cells (male and female)

11.7 There has been great excitement in this area with the generation of 'oocyte-like cells' from mouse embryonic stem cells.[88] Although confirmatory studies have yet to be published, there have been a number of reports showing 'oocyte-like cells' from a variety of other stem cell populations including fetal porcine skin[89] and rat adult pancreatic cells.[90] The ability of these cells to truly function as oocytes has yet to be established (meiotic competence, ability to form live young), but it is likely that oocyte-like cells will be produced for research purposes in the near future. At the same time this will further our understanding of what constitutes a germ cell. As exciting as this area is, it is unlikely that functional mature human eggs that can be used for clinical purposes will be derived from either adult or embryonic stem cells within the next five years.

11.8 Remarkably, progress for male germ cells has been even more rapid. Following reports of developing spermatids from spermatogonia *in vitro*,[91] functional sperm – generating live young – have been produced from mouse embryonic stem cells.[92] There are concerns over the health of the offspring as there were imprinting defects and much work is required to establish the repeatability and safety of this process. However, as our understanding of the culture conditions necessary to complete the critical stages of spermatogenesis *in vitro* continues to evolve rapidly[93] it is likely that haploid male gametes will be produced from human embryonic cells in the near future. However, functional mature human sperm that can be used for clinical purposes will not be available within the next five years.

Appendix 1

Useful organisations

General

Cancerbackup

3 Bath Place, Rivington Street, London EC2A 3JR

Tel: 0207 696 9003

Freephone 0808 800 1234 to speak to a cancer support service nurse, Monday–Friday, 9am–8pm

Email: info@cancerbackup.org

Website: www.cancerbackup.org.uk

Cancerbackup provides information, understanding and support for patients and their families on all types of cancer.

CancerIndex

Website: www.cancerindex.org

CancerIndex provides a guide to Internet resources for people suffering from cancer.

Cancer Research UK

P.O. Box 123, Lincoln's Inn Fields, London WC2A 3PX

Tel: 020 7242 0200

Freephone 0808 800 4040 to speak to a specialist nurse, Monday–Friday, 9am–5pm.

Website: www.cancerresearchuk.org

Cancer Research UK is the UK's leading cancer research charity. It also provides information and advice to patients and their families on its website CancerHelp UK (www.cancerhelp.org.uk).

Cancer in children and teenagers

UK Children's Cancer and Leukaemia Group (UKCCSG / UKCCLG)

University of Leicester, 3rd Floor, Hearts of Oak House, 9 Princess Road West, Leicester LE1 6TH

Tel: 0116 249 4460

Email: info@cclg.org.uk

Website: www.cclg.org.uk

CCLG is a national professional body responsible for the organisation of the treatment and management of children with cancer in the UK. It coordinates national and international clinical trials, including biological studies. Other areas of activity include national cancer registration and provision of information for patients and families. The UKCCSG has recently merged with the UK Childhood Leukaemia Working Party, and is now the UKCCLG.

The National Alliance of Childhood Cancer Parent Organisations (NACCPO)
Rachael Olley, Operations Manager, 23 Meadowbank Walk, Stafford ST16 1TA
or
NACCPO, PO Box 176, Bromley BR2 7YN
Tel: 01785 603 763
Email: ro@naccpo.org.uk
Website: www.naccpo.org.uk

NACCPO shares best practice between member local parent organisations in the UK and around the world, to support children with cancer. It aims to create a national voice for parents of children with cancer, by working with medical, government and charity organisations on a national level, to address issues affecting children with cancer and their families.

Teenage Cancer Trust (TCT)
3rd floor, 93 Newman Street, London W1T 3EZ
Tel: 0207 612 0370
Email: tct@teenagecancertrust.org
Website: www.teenagecancertrust.org

TCT focuses on the needs of teenagers and young adults with cancer, leukaemia, Hodgkin disease and related diseases by providing specialist teenage units in NHS hospitals. The units are dedicated areas for teenage patients, who are involved in their concept and creation.

Teen Info on Cancer (TIC)
Website: www.click4tic.org.uk

TIC's website, affiliated to Cancerbackup, provides information on cancer written for teenagers, advice and support on how to cope with cancer, and the space for teenagers to share their experiences of cancer with other teenagers.

Infertility, surrogacy and adoption

Human Fertilisation and Embryology Authority (HFEA)
21 Bloomsbury Street, London WC1B 3HF
Tel: 0207 291 8200
Email: admin@hfea.gov.uk
Website: www.hfea.gov.uk

The HFEA licenses and monitors UK clinics that offer IVF (in vitro fertilisation) and DI (donor insemination) treatments, and all UK-based research into human embryos. It also regulates the storage of eggs, sperm and embryos. It provides a range of information for patients, professionals and government.

British Fertility Society (BFS)
Sharon Phillips, BFS Secretariat, 22 Apex Court, Woodlands, Bradley Stoke BS32 4JT
Tel: 01454 642 277
Email: bfs@bioscientifica.com
Website: www.britishfertilitysociety.org.uk

The BFS provides a forum for members of disciplines with an interest in infertility, reproductive medicine and biology on practice, research, policy and ethics. It aims to promote high-quality practice, research and training; it also produces publications and liaises with professional, governmental and patient organisations.

Childlessness Overcome Through Surrogacy (COTS)
Moss Bank, Manse Road, Sutherland, Lairg IV27 4EL, Scotland
Tel: 01549 402 777
Email: info@surrogacy.org.uk
Website: www.surrogacy.org.uk

COTS is not a commercial agency. Its objective is to pass on collective experience to surrogates and would-be parents, helping them to understand the implications of surrogacy before they enter into an arrangement and to deal with any problems that may arise during it.

British Association for Adoption and Fostering (BAAF)
Saffron House, 6–10 Kirby Street, London EC1N 8TS
Tel: 020 7421 2600
Email: mail@baaf.org.uk
Website: www.baaf.org.uk

BAAF develops practice and policy guidelines for adoption and fostering as well as lobbying parliament and local government. It also provides assistance with child placement.

Overseas Adoption Support and Information Services (OASIS)
Helpline: 0870 241 7069
Email: membership@adoptionoverseas.org
Website: www.adoptionoverseas.org

OASIS is a UK-based voluntary support group for people who wish to adopt, or who have already adopted, children from orphanages overseas. It provides support and information from the first thoughts about overseas adoption, through the process itself and dealing with issues post adoption.

Association for Families who have Adopted from Abroad (AFAA)
30 Bradgate, Cuffley, Potters Bar, Herts EN6 4RL
Tel (Helpline): 01707 872129
Email: information.afaa@ntlworld.com
Website: www.afaa.org.uk

AFAA offers support to families who have adopted, or are considering adopting, children from abroad, and generally aims to promote inter-country adoption (ICA) as a well founded method of building a family.

Patient information on cancer treatment and fertility

Information for women

This information is about fertility (the ability to have children) and how it can sometimes be affected by cancer treatment. When you are diagnosed with cancer, your fertility may be important, although it may not be a priority for you at the time. For many women, however, fertility issues become increasingly relevant.

The information is written for women with cancer, and their partners. Separate information for men who have cancer is on pp 48–54.

We hope that this information will answer any questions that you have about this issue, so that you can plan for the future before your treatment starts. Obviously each individual's situation and concerns will be different, so **you should always feel free to ask questions and discuss things with your doctor or nurse at the hospital where you are having your treatment**.

We have included the following information:

- ▶ Your feelings
- ▶ Contraception during treatment
- ▶ What is fertility?
- ▶ Fertility in women
- ▶ Fertilisation
- ▶ How cancer treatment can affect fertility
- ▶ Preserving your fertility
- ▶ Are there any risks?
- ▶ Using donated eggs and sperm
- ▶ Hormone replacement therapy
- ▶ Further information and support
- ▶ Useful organisations

© Cancerbackup, Royal College of Physicians, The Royal College of Radiologists, Royal College of Obstetricians and Gynaecologists, 2007

* Health professionals may wish to tick the boxes beside the sections that they are advising individual patients to read.

* ☐ Your feelings

It may be that having cancer treatment has meant you have to think about your fertility sooner than you had planned. Or, fertility may always have been very important to you. Either way, to be told you have cancer and that the treatment may affect your fertility and could make you infertile can be very difficult.

For some women the possibility of losing their fertility can be as difficult to accept as the cancer diagnosis. But, for others beating the cancer is their only concern. There is no right or wrong way to feel and react.

The uncertainty surrounding fertility can make a very difficult time even harder. Don't be afraid to ask questions of your doctor or specialist nurse. They will be very happy to discuss things with you.

Everyone has their own way of coping with difficult situations and some people find it helpful to discuss how they are feeling with their partner, a close friend, or relative. It may also be possible to discuss how you are feeling with a specialist counsellor.

☐ Contraception during treatment

It's best to avoid getting pregnant during treatment with chemotherapy or radiotherapy. You should continue to use a reliable method of contraception for a period of time after treatment has finished, usually for at least a year, and your doctor or nurse can discuss this with you. With some types of cancer, for example breast cancer, it may not be advisable to take the oral contraceptive pill.

If you become pregnant during treatment you should tell your specialist or nurse as soon as possible, as there may be a risk to the health of a child conceived during treatment.

☐ What is fertility?

For women, fertility is the ability to get pregnant and it depends on having a supply of eggs from the ovaries. You are born with a large number of eggs and as you get older the number becomes fewer. When there are very few left, you go through the menopause (change of life).

☐ Fertility in women

To have a child, an egg from the woman needs to be fertilised by a sperm from a man. Once a month, from puberty to menopause, one of the ovaries produces and releases one of the eggs. The egg moves along the Fallopian tube to the womb, ready to be fertilised.

If the egg is fertilised by a sperm, the resulting embryo may bury itself in the lining of the womb and grow to form a baby. Hormones, which are the body's chemical messengers, are produced by the ovaries and these prepare the lining of the womb for the fertilised egg, so that it is ready to develop and maintain the pregnancy.

If the egg is not fertilised the woman will have a period.

☐ Fertilisation

Usually, sexual intercourse has to take place for the egg to be fertilised by a sperm. This involves the man achieving an erection and ejaculating sperm into the vagina. If this is not possible there are other, artificial or assisted, ways of fertilising an egg, which are described on page 44.

☐ How cancer treatment can affect fertility

Treatment for cancer can affect a woman's fertility in different ways. Some cancer treatments can:

- ▶ damage the ovaries, reducing the number of eggs available and causing an early menopause
- ▶ affect hormone production
- ▶ remove the womb
- ▶ damage the lining of the womb, making it difficult to maintain a pregnancy.

These treatment effects may make it impossible for fertilisation to take place normally through sex. In this situation it may be possible to use artificial or assisted methods to fertilise an egg in order to create an embryo (see page 44). Also, hormones can be replaced by hormone replacement therapy (HRT) (see page 46).

There are four main treatments for cancer and they can all affect fertility in some way:

- ▶ chemotherapy
- ▶ radiotherapy
- ▶ hormonal therapy
- ▶ surgery.

☐ *Chemotherapy*

Chemotherapy can often cause infertility. For most women this will be temporary; for others it will be permanent. The effect that chemotherapy has upon fertility – and whether it is temporary or permanent – will vary depending upon a number of factors. These include:

- ▶ the chemotherapy drugs used – some are more likely than others to cause a problem
- ▶ the dose of the drug used – higher doses are more likely to affect fertility
- ▶ whether a combination of chemotherapy drugs is given – a combination of drugs may be more likely to affect your fertility

▶ your age – the younger you are, the more likely you are to retain normal fertility

▶ your general health – your doctor or nurse will be able to discuss this with you further.

In some circumstances it may be possible to choose a chemotherapy treatment that is less likely to affect fertility. This may increase the chances of you recovering normal fertility after treatment.

Even when fertility returns after chemotherapy, your menopause may occur up to 10 or more years earlier than normally expected. This means that there might be a shorter time span than usual for trying to get pregnant and having a child.

☐ *Radiotherapy*

Radiotherapy given directly to the ovaries will cause permanent infertility. Radiotherapy that includes the womb can lead to infertility, and can also increase the risk of miscarriage and premature birth in women who do conceive.

The risk of infertility is generally related to the dose of radiotherapy given, and the risk increases if it is given in combination with chemotherapy. The risk of permanent infertility also increases with the age at which the person has treatment.

Total body irradiation (TBI) is given to some people with cancer and very often causes permanent infertility, although a small number of people who have this treatment will be able to have children afterwards.

Radioactive iodine, another form of radiotherapy, does not usually affect fertility.

Radiotherapy to the brain that includes the pituitary gland can sometimes affect the hormones that stimulate the ovaries to produce the female hormones, oestrogen and progesterone.

☐ *Hormonal therapy*

Some types of hormonal therapy may affect fertility. This effect is usually temporary and only lasts while the treatment is being taken.

☐ *Surgery*

Most operations for cancer do not affect your ability to get pregnant. However, some operations will mean that you will be unable to have a child. These are:

▶ having your womb removed (a hysterectomy)

▶ having both your ovaries removed (a bilateral oophorectomy)

▶ some types of surgery to the cervix, vulva and vagina.

Your surgeon or specialist nurse can give you more information about this.

☐ Preserving your fertility

It can be difficult to predict whether your fertility will be affected by cancer treatment or whether it will return to normal once the treatment has finished. Although some treatments for cancer may reduce fertility, it may still be possible to get pregnant once treatment has ended.

Women with a partner who are concerned that they may become infertile are advised to discuss storing embryos (fertilised eggs) for future use. This requires egg collection and fertilisation using sperm from a partner and will take 4–6 weeks. Embryos have been stored safely and successfully for many years, but it will not be possible without sperm and may not be advisable for some types of cancer.

Embryos can be frozen for up to ten years, although in some situations this can be extended. Your doctor or nurse can discuss this with you and can refer you to a fertility clinic before your cancer treatment starts. Sometimes the NHS will pay for storage of the embryos, but not always.

☐ *Egg collection*

The whole process of egg collection takes 4–6 weeks and involves stimulating the ovaries to produce more eggs than normal. This is done by giving injections of hormones. To increase the chances of achieving a pregnancy, as many eggs as possible are collected, usually at least six.

Eggs are normally collected using an ultrasound-guided needle which is passed through the wall of the vagina. This procedure can be uncomfortable and a local or general anaesthetic will be used.

Some women need to start their cancer treatment straightaway and it may not be possible to delay treatment in order to have ovarian stimulation.

There is a risk with some types of cancer, such as breast cancer, that the hormones used in ovarian stimulation may also make the cancer grow. Therefore it may not be advisable to have ovarian stimulation. Your doctors will be able to discuss this with you. It may be possible to collect one or two eggs without stimulation, although this reduces the chances of a successful pregnancy.

☐ *Embryo storage*

Once the eggs have been collected they can be fertilised using IVF (in vitro fertilisation) and then frozen. IVF involves putting your eggs together with sperm in a test tube in a laboratory for fertilisation to occur.

In order to fertilise the eggs to form an embryo, sperm from your partner is needed. Both of you must sign a consent form and neither can use the embryo to start a pregnancy without the other's permission. If you have no partner, sperm from a donor can be used (see page 45). When the embryos are needed, they are thawed and placed in the womb.

Large numbers of healthy babies have been born using this technique. Freezing embryos is not thought to increase the risk of abnormalities.

There may be a charge for IVF treatment in some areas of the UK. Your doctor, nurse or the staff at the fertility centre can discuss this with you.

☐ *Freezing unfertilised eggs*

This is a newer, more experimental technique. It is very much less successful than freezing embryos and so is not widely available. When the eggs are thawed they are fertilised by injecting a sperm into the egg. This is known as ICSI (intra-cytoplasmic sperm injection). The fertilised egg is then placed in the womb.

☐ *Ovarian tissue storage*

This type of infertility treatment is very experimental, and worldwide only a few babies have been born using this method. Small pieces of ovary (which contain eggs) are frozen and stored. Later the ovary tissue is put back into the body and any eggs which develop are collected.

Unfortunately, there are no guarantees of pregnancy with these treatments. If you have not been able to store any embryos, or eggs, or if you do not become pregnant by the above methods, it may be possible for you to use eggs from another woman (donor eggs) – see below.

If cancer treatment has damaged your ovaries but you manage to become pregnant by one of the methods listed here, it is likely that you will need to be given hormones to maintain the pregnancy. The hormones may be given by injection.

☐ Are there any risks?

If you get pregnant naturally after cancer treatment there are no increased risks of harm to the child.

The effect of radiotherapy and chemotherapy given to a woman before egg collection is not clear. There is a small theoretical possibility of damage to the child, but at the moment there is no evidence to suggest that children conceived using embryos stored after cancer treatment will be harmed in any way.

The use of stored embryos has been carried out for many years and it appears not to cause any increased risk of harm to the child. Newer techniques, such as ICSI, have been used less and the long-term risks to the children conceived using these methods are not fully known. At the moment the best information suggests the risks of harm are very small.

If you are concerned about the possible risks, it may help to discuss this with your doctor, specialist nurse, or the staff at the fertility clinic.

☐ Using donated eggs and sperm

If the cancer treatment has caused permanent infertility and you were unable to collect some of your eggs before your treatment, you may consider using donated eggs.

If you are able to collect eggs and would prefer to store embryos (rather than unfertilised eggs), but don't have a partner, it may be possible to use donated sperm.

Everyone who donates eggs or sperm is carefully selected. Usually an egg donor will be matched as closely as possible so that the eye and hair colour, physical build and ethnic origin are the same as the woman who can no longer produce eggs. Sperm donors will also be closely matched. The donor has to be fit and healthy with no medical problems and will be tested for various infectious diseases. There is a shortage of egg donors in the UK, so you may have to wait to find a suitable donor.

Choosing to use donated eggs or sperm is a difficult decision and will often need very careful consideration. It isn't going to suit everyone. The staff at the fertility clinic, your doctors and specialist nurse can discuss this with you further.

☐ Hormone replacement therapy

If you have an early menopause as a result of cancer treatment, you may be offered hormone replacement therapy (HRT). HRT can help to prevent problems associated with the menopause, such as thinning of the bones (osteoporosis) and heart disease. However, HRT isn't recommended if you have had certain types of cancer, such as breast cancer. Your doctor can discuss this with you further.

Some women regain their fertility after HRT has begun, so if you don't want to get pregnant it is advisable to also use reliable methods of contraception, or to take the oral contraceptive pill instead of having HRT. The pill will replace your hormones and also prevent pregnancy. Again, you can discuss this in more detail with your doctor.

☐ Further information and support

Many hospitals have specialist nurses who may be able to help you. Some hospitals and fertility clinics also have fertility counsellors who you could talk to.

You may also want to discuss this information with one of the cancer support services nurses on Cancerbackup's freephone helpline 0808 800 1234. Lines are open Monday–Friday, 9–8pm (an interpreting service is available).

Cancerbackup is the UK's leading cancer information charity, providing information, understanding and support on any cancer via: 70 booklets and over 300 factsheets free direct to patients and their families; its comprehensive website (www.cancerbackup.org.uk); eight walk-in information centres in England; and its helpline. All of Cancerbackup's information is also available online at www.cancerbackup.org.uk

You could also contact one of the support organisations listed on page 47.

☐ Useful organisations

Cancer Research UK

PO Box 123, Lincoln's Inn Fields,
London WC2A 3PX
Website: www.cancerhelp.org.uk
Tel: 020 7061 8355
Freephone 0808 800 4040
to speak to a specialist nurse,
Monday–Friday, 9am–5pm.

The UK's leading cancer research charity.
CancerHelp UK is one of its five main websites and
provides a comprehensive free information service
about cancer and cancer care for people with cancer
and their families.

British Infertility Counselling Association

111 Harley Street, London, W1G 6AW
Website: http://74.220.203.213/bica/index.php

A charity dedicated to providing the highest standard
of counselling and support to people affected by
infertility. The website can be used to find a counsellor
in your area.

Human Fertilisation and Embryology Authority (HFEA)

21 Bloomsbury Street, London, WC1B 3HF
Tel: 020 7291 8200
Fax: 020 7291 8201
Email: admin@hfea.gov.uk
Website: www.hfea.gov.uk

A government body responsible for licensing fertility
treatment centres and for maintaining a code of
practice. They also regulate donor information and
monitor fertility research. They hold a list of all the
fertility clinics in the UK.

Infertility Ireland

National Infertility Support and Information Group
PO Box 131, Togher, Cork, Ireland
Tel: 1890 647 444 (Lo-call)
Email: nisig@eircom.net
Website: www.infertilityireland.ie

A voluntary organisation that offers support and
information to people affected by infertility.

Infertility Network UK

Charter House, 43 St Leonards Road,
Bexhill on Sea, TN40 1JA
Tel: 08701 188 088
Email: admin@infertilitynetworkuk.com
Website: www.infertilitynetworkuk.com

A national support network for people with infertility,
provided through national and regional offices covering
the whole of the UK. Information, advice and
counselling is available covering all aspects of infertility.

Teen Info on Cancer (TIC)

www.click4tic.org.uk

A website for young/teenage cancer patients. Affiliated
to Cancerbackup, it provides links to information and
advice on cancer.

The National Alliance of Childhood Cancer Parent Organisations (NACCPO)

Rachael Olley, Operations Manager,
23 Meadowbank Walk, Stafford ST16 1TA
or
NACCPO, PO Box 176, Bromley BR2 7YN
Tel: 01785 603 763
Email: ro@naccpo.org.uk
Website: www.naccpo.org.uk

Parent-run organisations with common aims of working
together to support children with cancer, sharing best
practice between local parent organisations in the UK
and around the world.

Related Cancerbackup information

- ▶ Relationships, Sex and Fertility for Young People Affected by Cancer
- ▶ Sexuality and Cancer
- ▶ The Emotional Effects of Cancer

For copies of this related information call free on 0808
800 1234, or see it online at www.cancerbackup.org.uk

This information has been produced as a collaboration between
Cancerbackup and a Working Party of the Royal College of
Physicians, The Royal College of Radiologists and the Royal
College of Obstetricians and Gynaecologists.

© Cancerbackup, Royal College of Physicians, The Royal College
of Radiologists, Royal College of Obstetricians and
Gynaecologists, 2007

Patient information on cancer treatment and fertility

Information for men

This information is about fertility (the ability to have children) and how it may sometimes be affected by cancer treatment. When you are diagnosed with cancer, your fertility may be important, although it may not be a priority for you at the time. For many men, however, fertility issues become increasingly relevant.

This information is written for men with cancer, and their partners. Separate information for women who have cancer is on pp 40–47.

We hope that this information will answer any questions that you have about this issue, so that you can plan for the future before your treatment starts. Obviously each individual's situation and concerns will be different, so **you should always feel free to ask questions and discuss things with your doctor or nurse at the hospital where you are having your treatment.**

We have included the following information:

- ▶ Your feelings
- ▶ Contraception during treatment
- ▶ Fertility in men
- ▶ How cancer treatment can affect fertility
- ▶ Preserving your fertility
- ▶ Are there any risks?
- ▶ Using donated sperm
- ▶ Testosterone replacement therapy
- ▶ Further information and support
- ▶ Useful organisations

© Cancerbackup, Royal College of Physicians, The Royal College of Radiologists, Royal College of Obstetricians and Gynaecologists, 2007

* Health professionals may wish to tick the boxes beside the sections that they are advising individual patients to read.

* ☐ Your feelings

To be told that you have cancer and that treatment may affect your fertility, and could make you infertile, can be very difficult. For some men, the threat of losing their fertility can be as difficult to accept as the cancer diagnosis. For other men, beating the cancer is their only concern. There is no right or wrong way to feel and react.

The uncertainty surrounding fertility can make a very difficult time even harder. Don't be afraid to ask questions of your doctor or specialist nurse. They will be very happy to discuss things with you.

Everyone has their own way of coping with difficult situations and some people find it helpful to discuss how they are feeling with their partner, a close friend, or relative. It may also be possible to discuss how you are feeling with a specialist counsellor.

☐ Contraception during treatment

During the time you are being treated with chemotherapy or radiotherapy, it is best to avoid getting your partner pregnant. There is an unproven possibility that chemotherapy might damage your sperm and could therefore damage the health of a baby conceived during that time. You should continue to use contraception after treatment, usually for at least a year, and your doctor or nurse can discuss this with you.

☐ Fertility in men

From puberty onwards the testicles begin to produce sperm, millions at a time. They are stored in the testicles until needed. The production of sperm is controlled by various hormones, which are the body's chemical messengers. Hormones also control sex drive and the ability to get an erection.

Usually, sexual intercourse has to take place for a woman's egg to be fertilised by a male sperm. This involves the man getting an erection and ejaculating sperm into a woman's vagina. For this to happen, the nerves and blood vessels in the pelvic area and genitals need to be working normally.

So normal fertility in men (ie the ability to get a woman pregnant) depends on both active sperm in the testicles and the ability to have an erection, penetrate the vagina and ejaculate. The sperm can then be released and fertilise the woman's egg.

It is important to know that being able to get an erection and ejaculate does not always mean that you are fertile. You might be producing too few sperm or none at all. Some cancer treatments affect only sperm production, so intercourse can still take place. Other treatments can affect the ability to get an erection and ejaculate, but normal sperm might still be produced.

If sexual intercourse isn't possible there are other, artificial or assisted, ways of fertilising an egg, which are described on pages 51–52.

☐ How cancer treatment can affect fertility

Treatments for cancer can affect a man's fertility in different ways. Some cancer treatments can:

- ▶ stop the production of sperm (temporarily or permanently)
- ▶ affect the production of the hormone testosterone, which can influence your sex drive and your ability to get an erection
- ▶ damage the nerves and blood vessels in the pelvic area, which can affect your ability to get an erection and/or ejaculate normally.

These treatment effects may make it impossible for fertilisation to take place normally through sex. In this situation there are artificial methods of using sperm to fertilise eggs to create an embryo (see page 52). Also, testosterone can be replaced by testosterone replacement therapy (see page 53).

There are four main treatments for cancer and they can all affect fertility in some way:

- ▶ chemotherapy
- ▶ radiotherapy
- ▶ hormonal therapy
- ▶ surgery.

☐ Chemotherapy

Chemotherapy can often cause infertility by affecting sperm production. For most men this will be temporary; for others it will be permanent. The effect that chemotherapy has upon fertility – and whether it is temporary or permanent – will vary depending upon a number of factors. These include:

- ▶ the chemotherapy drugs used – as some are more likely than others to cause a problem
- ▶ the dose of the drug used – higher doses are more likely to affect fertility
- ▶ whether a combination of chemotherapy drugs is given – a combination of drugs may be more likely to affect fertility
- ▶ your general health – your doctor or nurse will be able to discuss this with you further.

It may be possible in some circumstances to choose a chemotherapy treatment that is less likely to affect your fertility. This may increase the chances of you recovering normal fertility after treatment.

After chemotherapy it might take two years or more for your normal fertility to return. Sexual functioning (erection and ejaculation) should not be affected.

☐ Radiotherapy

Radiotherapy given directly to the testicles will cause permanent infertility by stopping sperm production. Radiotherapy given to the pelvic area can also lead to reduced sperm production, which may be temporary or permanent.

The risk of infertility is generally related to the dose of radiotherapy given. A return to normal sperm production may take up to five years. If sperm have not returned after this length of time, they are unlikely to return at all.

Total body irradiation (TBI) is given to some people with cancer, and usually causes permanent infertility, although a small number of people who have this treatment will be able to have children afterwards.

Radioactive iodine, another form of radiotherapy, does not usually affect fertility.

Radiotherapy to the brain that includes the pituitary gland can sometimes affect the hormones that stimulate the testicles to produce testosterone. Radiotherapy to the testicles can also reduce the amount of testosterone that is produced. A lack of testosterone can reduce sex drive and the ability to get an erection.

☐ *Hormonal therapy*

Some types of hormonal therapy may affect fertility. Generally this effect will be temporary and only lasts for the duration of the treatment.

☐ *Surgery*

Most operations for cancer do not affect your ability to get your partner pregnant. However, some operations will mean that you will be unable to have a child. Having both testicles removed (a bilateral orchidectomy) will mean that you will not be able to father children. Having one testicle removed should not affect your ability to have children, as the remaining testicle will usually function normally.

Some types of surgery to the pelvic area or to the spine may make you unable to have sexual intercourse because they can damage the nerves and blood vessels in the pelvic area, making it impossible to get an erection.

☐ Preserving your fertility

It can be difficult to predict whether your fertility will be affected by cancer treatment or whether it will return to normal once the treatment has finished. Although some treatments for cancer may reduce fertility, it may still be possible to father a child once treatment has ended.

Many men and boys are advised to discuss storing sperm for future use. Sperm storage is a safe technique that has been successfully carried out for many years.

Samples of sperm are frozen until needed and can be kept in storage until you reach 55. Your doctor or nurse can discuss this with you and can refer you to a fertility clinic before your cancer treatment starts. Sometimes treatment may need to start straightaway and sperm collection may not be possible. Sometimes the NHS will pay for the storage of sperm for men affected by cancer, but not always.

☐ *Collection of sperm*

Usually you will be asked to produce a sperm sample by masturbation in the fertility clinic. Some men find it difficult and embarrassing to produce a sperm sample in this way. The staff at the fertility clinic will try to make things as easy as possible for you and maintain your privacy at all times. In some circumstances it may be possible to bring a sample in from home as long as you can do this within 30–45 minutes and the appropriate consent has been signed.

Before the samples are stored you will have to sign a consent form that states how the sperm is to be used. Sperm storage is generally not advised once chemotherapy has begun.

You will be asked to provide two or three sperm samples for storage, which are collected over the course of about a week. It is advisable not to have sexual activity for a couple of days before collecting each sample. This helps to ensure that each sample contains enough sperm that are healthy and can fertilise an egg.

Previously, large numbers of sperm were required to fertilise an egg. However, a newer technique known as ICSI (intra-cytoplasmic sperm injection) can sometimes be used. This involves injecting a single sperm into the egg. This means that even samples containing low numbers of sperm, of any quality, are worth freezing. This is helpful when treatment needs to be started quickly, or if the sperm is of poor quality because of the effect of the cancer.

If you are unable to produce samples, or if the sample is inadequate, it may be possible to look for sperm by removing a piece of testicular tissue. The doctor or nurse at the fertility clinic can give you more information about this.

Unfortunately, there are no guarantees that stored sperm will be able to fertilise an egg and achieve a pregnancy. This will be discussed with you at the clinic before storage. If you are not able to store sperm or the sperm does not achieve a pregnancy, it may be possible for your partner to use sperm from another man (donated sperm); see page 53.

☐ Are there any risks?

If you father a child normally after cancer treatment there are no increased risks of harm to the child.

The use of stored sperm has been carried out for many years and it appears not to cause any increased risk of harm to the child. Newer techniques, such as ICSI, have been used much less and the long-term risks to children conceived using these methods are not fully known. At the moment the best information suggests the risks of harm are very small.

The effect of radiotherapy and chemotherapy before sperm storage is not clear. There is a small theoretical possibility of damage to the child, but at the moment there is no evidence to suggest that children conceived using sperm stored after cancer treatment will be harmed in any way.

If you are concerned about the possible risks, it may help to discuss this with your doctor, specialist nurse, or the staff at the fertility clinic.

☐ Using donated sperm

If the cancer treatment has caused permanent infertility and you were unable to store sperm, you and your partner may consider using donated sperm.

Everyone who donates sperm is carefully selected. Usually a donor will be matched as closely as possible so that the eye and hair colour, physical build and ethnic origin are the same as the man who can no longer produce sperm. The donor has to be fit and healthy with no medical problems and will be tested for various infectious diseases.

Choosing to use donated sperm is a difficult decision and will often need very careful consideration. It isn't going to suit everyone. The staff at the fertility clinic, your doctors and specialist nurse can discuss this with you further.

There is a shortage of sperm donors in the UK so you may have to wait to find a suitable donor.

☐ Testosterone replacement therapy

If you have had radiotherapy to the pituitary gland in the brain, or to the testicles, you may have reduced levels of testosterone. This can happen many years after treatment. A lack of testosterone can affect your ability to get an erection and reduce your sex drive. It can also affect your health, and can cause problems such as thinning of the bones (osteoporosis).

Testosterone replacement therapy will help to reduce these problems. Replacement therapy will be given for life. It can be given as a patch that is stuck on the skin (transdermal), as an implant or as an injection into a muscle. Your doctor can give you more advice about testosterone replacement therapy.

☐ Further information and support

Many hospitals have specialist nurses who may be able to help you. Some hospitals and fertility clinics also have fertility counsellors that you could talk to.

You may also want to discuss this information with one of the cancer support services nurses on Cancerbackup's freephone helpline 0808 800 1234. Lines are open Monday–Friday, 9am–8pm (an interpreting service is available).

Cancerbackup is the UK's leading cancer information charity, providing information, understanding and support on any cancer via: 70 booklets and over 300 factsheets free direct to patients and their families; its comprehensive website (www.cancerbackup.org.uk); eight walk-in information centres in England; and its helpline. All of Cancerbackup's information is also available online at www.cancerbackup.org.uk

You could also contact one of the support organisations listed on page 54.

☐   Useful organisations

Cancer Research UK

PO Box 123, Lincoln's Inn Fields,
London WC2A 3PX
Website: www.cancerhelp.org.uk
Tel: 020 7061 8355
Freephone 0808 800 4040
to speak to a specialist nurse,
Monday–Friday, 9am–5pm.

The UK's leading cancer research charity.
CancerHelp UK is one of its five main websites and
provides a comprehensive free information service
about cancer and cancer care for people with cancer
and their families.

British Infertility Counselling Association

111 Harley Street, London, W1G 6AW
Website: http://74.220.203.213/bica/index.php

A charity dedicated to providing the highest standard
of counselling and support to people affected by
infertility. The website can be used to find a counsellor
in your area.

Human Fertilisation and Embryology Authority (HFEA)

21 Bloomsbury Street, London, WC1B 3HF
Tel: 020 7291 8200
Fax: 020 7291 8201
Email: admin@hfea.gov.uk
Website: www.hfea.gov.uk

A government body responsible for licensing fertility
treatment centres and for maintaining a code of
practice. They also regulate donor information and
monitor fertility research. They hold a list of all the
fertility clinics in the UK.

Infertility Ireland

National Infertility Support and Information Group
PO Box 131, Togher, Cork, Ireland
Tel: 1890 647 444 (Lo-call)
Email: nisig@eircom.net
Website: www.infertilityireland.ie

A voluntary organisation that offers support and
information to people affected by infertility.

Infertility Network UK

Charter House, 43 St Leonards Road,
Bexhill on Sea, TN40 1JA
Tel: 08701 188 088
Email: admin@infertilitynetworkuk.com
Website: www.infertilitynetworkuk.com

A national support network for people with infertility,
provided through national and regional offices covering
the whole of the UK. Information, advice and
counselling is available covering all aspects of infertility.

Teen Info on Cancer (TIC)

www.click4tic.org.uk

A website for young/teenage cancer patients. Affiliated
to Cancerbackup, it provides links to information and
advice on cancer.

The National Alliance of Childhood Cancer Parent Organisations (NACCPO)

Rachael Olley, Operations Manager,
23 Meadowbank Walk, Stafford ST16 1TA
or
NACCPO, PO Box 176, Bromley BR2 7YN
Tel: 01785 603 763
Email: ro@naccpo.org.uk
Website: www.naccpo.org.uk

Parent-run organisations with common aims of working
together to support children with cancer, sharing best
practice between local parent organisations in the UK
and around the world.

Related Cancerbackup information

- ▶ Relationships, Sex and Fertility for Young People Affected by Cancer
- ▶ Sexuality and Cancer
- ▶ The Emotional Effects of Cancer

For copies of this related information call free on 0808
800 1234, or see it online at www.cancerbackup.org.uk

This information has been produced as a collaboration between
Cancerbackup and a Working Party of the Royal College of
Physicians, The Royal College of Radiologists and the Royal
College of Obstetricians and Gynaecologists.

© Cancerbackup, Royal College of Physicians, The Royal College
of Radiologists, Royal College of Obstetricians and
Gynaecologists, 2007

References

1 Lobo RA. Potential options for preservation of fertility in women. *N Engl J Med* 2005;353:64–73.

2 Lee SJ, Schover LR, Partridge AH *et al*. American Society of Clinical Oncology recommendations on fertility preservation in cancer patients. *J Clin Oncol* 2006;24:2917–31.

3 Cancer Research UK. www.info.cancerresearchuk.org/cancerstats/incidence/. Accessed 5 Feb 2007.

4 Royal College of Physicians. *Management of gonadal toxicity resulting from the treatment of adult cancer*. Report of a working party of the Joint Council for Clinical Oncology. London: RCP, 1998.

5 World Health Organization. *WHO laboratory manual for the examination of human semen and sperm-cervical mucus interaction*, 4th edn. Cambridge: Cambridge University Press,1999.

6 Osmanagaoglu K, Vernaeve V, Kolibianakis E *et al*. Cumulative delivery rates after ICSI treatment cycles with freshly retrieved testicular sperm: a 7-year follow-up study. *Hum Reprod* 2003;18:1836–40.

7 Lutchman Singh K, Davies M, Chatterjee R. Fertility in female cancer survivors: pathophysiology, preservation and the role of ovarian reserve testing. *Hum Reprod Update* 2005;11:69–89.

8 Sonmezer M, Oktay K. Fertility preservation in female patients. *Hum Reprod Update* 2004;10:251–66.

9 Anderson RA, Themmen APN, Al Qahtani A *et al*. The effects of chemotherapy and long-term gonadotrophin suppression on the ovarian reserve in premenopausal women with breast cancer. *Human Reprod* 2006;21:2583–92.

10 Howell SJ, Shalet SM. Spermatogenesis after cancer treatment: damage and recovery. *J Natl Cancer Inst Monogr* 2005;34:12–7.

11 Kubo H, Shipley WU. Reduction of the scatter dose to the testicle outside the radiation treatment fields. *Int J Radiat Oncol Biol Phys* 1982;8:1741–5.

12 Hahn EW, Feingold SM, Simpson L, Batata M. Recovery from aspermia induced by low-dose radiation in seminoma patients. *Cancer* 1982;50:337–40.

13 Wallace WH, Thomson AB, Saran F, Kelsey TW. Predicting age of ovarian failure after radiation to a field that includes the ovaries. *Int J Radiat Oncol Biol Phys* 2005;62:738–44.

14 Mazonakis M, Damilakis J, Varveris H, Gourtsoyiannis N. Radiation dose to laterally transposed ovaries during external beam radiotherapy for cervical cancer. *Acta Oncol* 2006;45:702–7.

15 Urbano MT, Tait DM. Can the irradiated uterus sustain a pregnancy? A literature review. *Clin Oncol (R Coll Radiol)* 2004;16:24–8.

16 Critchley HO, Wallace WH. Impact of cancer treatment on uterine function. *J Natl Cancer Inst Monogr* 2005;34:64–8.

17 Schimmer AD, Quatermain M, Imrie K *et al*. Ovarian function after autologous bone marrow transplantation. *J Clin Oncol* 1998;16:2359–63.

18 Hyer S, Vini L, O'Connell M *et al*. Testicular dose and fertility in men following I(131) therapy for thyroid cancer. *Clin Endocrinol (Oxf)* 2002;56:755–8.

19 Chow SM, Yau S, Lee SH *et al*. Pregnancy outcome after diagnosis of differentiated thyroid carcinoma: no deleterious effect after radioactive iodine treatment. *Int J Radiat Oncol Biol Phys* 2004;59:992–1000.

20 Bal C, Kumar A, Tripathi M *et al.* High-dose radioiodine treatment for differentiated thyroid carcinoma is not associated with change in female fertility or any genetic risk to the offspring. *Int J Radiat Oncol Biol Phys* 2005;63:449–55.

21 Ceccarelli C, Battisti P, Gasperi M *et al.* Radiation dose to the testes after 131I therapy for ablation of postsurgical thyroid remnants in patients with differentiated thyroid cancer. *J Nucl Med* 1999;40:1716–21.

22 Early Breast Cancer Trialists' Collaborative Group (EBCTCG). Effects of chemotherapy and hormonal therapy for early breast cancer on recurrence and 15-year survival: an overview of the randomised trials. *Lancet* 2005;365:1687–717.

23 Brown RJ, Davidson NE. Adjuvant hormonal therapy for premenopausal women with breast cancer. *Semin Oncol* 2006;33:657–63.

24 Seidman AD. Systemic treatment of breast cancer. Two decades of progress. *Oncology (Williston Park)* 2006;20:983–90; discussion 991–2, 997–8.

25 Meric-Bernstam F, Hung MC. Advances in targeting human epidermal growth factor receptor-2 signaling for cancer therapy. *Clin Cancer Res* 2006;12:6326–30.

26 Molina JR, Barton DL, Loprinzi CL. Chemotherapy-induced ovarian failure: manifestations and management. *Drug Saf* 2005;28:401–16.

27 Walshe JM, Denduluri N, Swain SM. Amenorrhea in premenopausal women after adjuvant chemotherapy for breast cancer. *J Clin Oncol* 2006;24:5769–79.

28 Ganz PA. Breast cancer, menopause, and long-term survivorship: critical issues for the 21st century. *Am J Med* 2005;118(Suppl 12B):136–41.

29 Somers EC, Marder W, Christman GM *et al.* Use of a gonadotropin-releasing hormone analog for protection against premature ovarian failure during cyclophosphamide therapy in women with severe lupus. *Arthritis Rheum* 2005;52:2761–7.

30 Oktay K. Further evidence on the safety and success of ovarian stimulation with letrozole and tamoxifen in breast cancer patients undergoing in vitro fertilization to cryopreserve their embryos for fertility preservation. *J Clin Oncol* 2005;23:3858–9.

31 Beck JI, Boothroyd C, Proctor M *et al.* Oral anti-oestrogens and medical adjuncts for subfertility associated with anovulation. *Cochrane Database Syst Rev* 2005:CD002249.

32 Adelson KB, Loprinzi CL, Hershman DL. Treatment of hot flushes in breast and prostate cancer. *Expert Opin Pharmacother* 2005;6:1095–106.

33 Hickey M, Saunders CM, Stuckey BG. Management of menopausal symptoms in patients with breast cancer: an evidence-based approach. *Lancet Oncol* 2005;6:687–95.

34 Kroiss R, Fentiman IS, Helmond FA *et al.* The effect of tibolone in postmenopausal women receiving tamoxifen after surgery for breast cancer: a randomised, double-blind, placebo-controlled trial. *BJOG* 2005;112:228–33.

35 Loibl S, von Minckwitz G, Gwyn K *et al.* Breast carcinoma during pregnancy. International recommendations from an expert meeting. *Cancer* 2006;106:237–46.

36 Ives A, Saunders C, Bulsara M, Semmens J. Pregnancy after breast cancer: population based study. *BMJ* 2007;334:194–8.

37 Petersen PM, Skakkebaek NE, Rorth M, Giwercman A. Semen quality and reproductive hormones before and after orchiectomy in men with testicular cancer. *J Urol* 1999;161:822–6.

38 Brydoy M, Fossa SD, Klepp O *et al.* Paternity following treatment for testicular cancer. *J Natl Cancer Inst* 2005;97:1580–8.

39 Huddart RA, Norman A, Moynihan C *et al.* Fertility, gonadal and sexual function in survivors of testicular cancer. *Br J Cancer* 2005;93:200–7.

40 Petersen PM, Giwercman A, Hansen SW *et al.* Impaired testicular function in patients with carcinoma-in-situ of the testis. *J Clin Oncol* 1999;17:173–9.

41 Fossa SD, Horwich A, Russell JM *et al.* Optimal planning target volume for stage I testicular seminoma: a Medical Research Council randomized trial. Medical Research Council Testicular Tumor Working Group. *J Clin Oncol* 1999;17:1146.

42 Petersen PM, Giwercman A, Daugaard G *et al.* Effect of graded testicular doses of radiotherapy in patients treated for carcinoma-in-situ in the testis. *J Clin Oncol* 2002;20:1537–43.

43 Oliver RT, Mason MD, Mead GM *et al.* Radiotherapy versus single-dose carboplatin in adjuvant treatment of stage I seminoma: a randomised trial. *Lancet* 2005;366:293–300.

44 Petersen PM, Skakkebaek NE, Vistisen K *et al.* Semen quality and reproductive hormones before orchiectomy in men with testicular cancer. *J Clin Oncol* 1999;17:941–7.

45 Chan PT, Palermo GD, Veeck LL *et al.* Testicular sperm extraction combined with intracytoplasmic sperm injection in the treatment of men with persistent azoospermia postchemotherapy. *Cancer* 2001;92:1632–7.

46 Nuver J, Smit AJ, Wolffenbuttel BH *et al.* The metabolic syndrome and disturbances in hormone levels in long-term survivors of disseminated testicular cancer. *J Clin Oncol* 2005;23:3718–25.

47 Cancer Research UK. www.info.cancerresearchuk.org/cancerstats/types/cervix/incidence/. Accessed 6 Feb 2007.

48 Clough KB, Goffinet F, Labib A *et al.* Laparoscopic unilateral ovarian transposition prior to irradiation: prospective study of 20 cases. *Cancer* 1996;77:2638–45.

49 Dargent D, Martin X, Sacchetoni A, Mathevet P. Laparoscopic vaginal radical trachelectomy: a treatment to preserve the fertility of cervical carcinoma patients. *Cancer* 2000;88:1877–82.

50 Boss EA, van Golde RJ, Beerendonk CC, Massuger LF. Pregnancy after radical trachelectomy: a real option? *Gynecol Oncol* 2005;99:S152–6.

51 Whelan JS, Cassoni AM, Pollock R. Bone. In: Price P, Sikora K (eds), *Treatment of cancer*, 5th edn. London: Chapman and Hall, in press.

52 Kreuser ED, Hetzel WD, Heit W *et al.* Reproductive and endocrine gonadal functions in adults following multidrug chemotherapy for acute lymphoblastic or undifferentiated leukemia. *J Clin Oncol* 1988;6:588–95.

53 Salooja N, Szydlo RM, Socie G *et al.* Pregnancy outcomes after peripheral blood or bone marrow transplantation: a retrospective survey. *Lancet* 2001;358:271–6.

54 Sanders JE, Hawley J, Levy W *et al.* Pregnancies following high-dose cyclophosphamide with or without high-dose busulfan or total-body irradiation and bone marrow transplantation. *Blood* 1996;87:3045–52.

55 Rovo A, Tichelli A, Passweg JR *et al.* Spermatogenesis in long-term survivors after allogeneic hematopoietic stem cell transplantation is associated with age, time interval since transplantation, and apparently absence of chronic GvHD. *Blood* 2006;108:1100–5.

56 Royal College of Obstetricians and Gynaecologists. *Storage of ovarian and prepubertal testicular tissue.* Report of a working party. London: RCOG Press, 2000.

57 British Fertility Society. A strategy for fertility services for survivors of childhood cancer. *Hum Fertil* 2003;6:A1–A40.

58   Oktay K, Hourvitz A, Sahin G *et al.* Letrozole reduces estrogen and gonadotropin exposure in women with breast cancer undergoing ovarian stimulation before chemotherapy. *J Clin Endocrinol Metab* 2006;91:3885–90.

59   Donnez J, Martinez-Madrid B, Jadoul P *et al.* Ovarian tissue cryopreservation and transplantation: a review. *Hum Reprod Update* 2006;12:519–35.

60   Bonduelle M, Wennerholm UB, Loft A *et al.* A multi-centre cohort study of the physical health of 5-year-old children conceived after intracytoplasmic sperm injection, in vitro fertilization and natural conception. *Hum Reprod* 2005;20:413–9.

61   Lie RT, Lyngstadaas A, Orstavik KH *et al.* Birth defects in children conceived by ICSI compared with children conceived by other IVF-methods; a meta-analysis. *Int J Epidemiol* 2005;34:696–701.

62   47th Royal College of Obstetricians and Gynaecologists Study Group. *Menopause and hormone replacement.* RCOG: London; 2004.

63   Howell SJ, Radford JA, Ryder WD, Shalet SM. Testicular function after cytotoxic chemotherapy: evidence of Leydig cell insufficiency. *J Clin Oncol* 1999;17:1493–8.

64   Nieschlag E, Behre HM, Bouchard P *et al.* Testosterone replacement therapy: current trends and future directions. *Hum Reprod Update* 2004;10:409–19.

65   Morales A. Monitoring androgen replacement therapy: testosterone and prostate safety. *J Endocrinol Invest* 2005;28:122–7.

66   Kirshon B, Wasserstrum N, Willis R *et al.* Teratogenic effects of first-trimester cyclophosphamide therapy. *Obstet Gynecol* 1988;72:462–4.

67   Meirow D, Schiff E. Appraisal of chemotherapy effects on reproductive outcome according to animal studies and clinical data. *J Natl Cancer Inst Monogr* 2005;34:21–5.

68   Rostom AY, O'Cathail S. Failure of lactation following radiotherapy for breast cancer. *Lancet* 1986;1:163–4.

69   Sorensen K, Levitt G, Sebag-Montefiore D *et al.* Cardiac function in Wilms' tumor survivors. *J Clin Oncol* 1995;13:1546–56.

70   Lipshultz SE, Colan SD, Gelber RD *et al.* Late cardiac effects of doxorubicin therapy for acute lymphoblastic leukemia in childhood. *N Engl J Med* 1991;324:808–15.

71   Davis LE, Brown CE. Peripartum heart failure in a patient treated previously with doxorubicin. *Obstet Gynecol* 1988;71:506–8.

72   Levitt GA, Jenney ME. The reproductive system after childhood cancer. *Br J Obstet Gynaecol* 1998;105:946–53.

73   Critchley HOD, Bath LE, Wallace WHB. Radiation damage to the uterus — review of the effects of treatment of childhood cancer. *Hum Fertil (Camb)* 2002;5:61–6.

74   Green DM, Whitton JA, Stovall M *et al.* Pregnancy outcome of female survivors of childhood cancer: a report from the Childhood Cancer Survivor Study. *Am J Obstet Gynecol* 2002;187:1070–80.

75   Hawkins MM. Pregnancy outcome and offspring after childhood cancer. *BMJ* 1994;309:1034.

76   Li FP, Gimbrere K, Gelber RD *et al.* Outcome of pregnancy in survivors of Wilms' tumor. *JAMA* 1987;257:216–9.

77   Holmes GE, Holmes FF. Pregnancy outcome of patients treated for Hodgkin's disease: a controlled study. *Cancer* 1978;41:1317–22.

78   Hawkins MM, Draper GJ, Winter DL. Cancer in the offspring of survivors of childhood leukaemia and non-Hodgkin lymphomas. *Br J Cancer* 1995;71:1335–9.

79   Orwig KE, Schlatt S. Cryopreservation and transplantation of spermatogonia and testicular tissue for preservation of male fertility. *J Natl Cancer Inst Monogr* 2005:51–6.

80   Shinohara T, Kato M, Takehashi M *et al.* Rats produced by interspecies spermatogonial transplantation in mice and in vitro microinsemination. *Proc Natl Acad Sci USA* 2006;103:13624–8.

81   Oktay K, Cil AP, Bang H. Efficiency of oocyte cryopreservation: a meta-analysis. *Fertil Steril* 2006;86:70–80.

82   Chen SU, Lien YR, Chen HF *et al.* Observational clinical follow-up of oocyte cryopreservation using a slow-freezing method with 1,2-propanediol plus sucrose followed by ICSI. *Hum Reprod* 2005;20:1975–80.

83   Soderstrom-Anttila V, Makinen S, Tuuri T, Suikkari AM. Favourable pregnancy results with insemination of in vitro matured oocytes from unstimulated patients. *Hum Reprod* 2005;20:1534–40.

84   Soderstrom-Anttila V, Salokorpi T, Pihlaja M *et al.* Obstetric and perinatal outcome and preliminary results of development of children born after in vitro maturation of oocytes. *Hum Reprod* 2006;21:1508–13.

85   Oktay K, Buyuk E, Veeck L *et al.* Embryo development after heterotopic transplantation of cryopreserved ovarian tissue. *Lancet* 2004;363:837–40.

86   O'Brien MJ, Pendola JK, Eppig JJ. A revised protocol for in vitro development of mouse oocytes from primordial follicles dramatically improves their developmental competence. *Biol Reprod* 2003;68:1682–6.

87   Wu D, Cheung QC, Wen L, Li J. A growth-maturation system that enhances the meiotic and developmental competence of porcine oocytes isolated from small follicles. *Biol Reprod* 2006;75:547–54.

88   Hubner K, Fuhrmann G, Christenson LK *et al.* Derivation of oocytes from mouse embryonic stem cells. *Science* 2003;300:1251–6.

89   Dyce PW, Wen L, Li J. In vitro germline potential of stem cells derived from fetal porcine skin. *Nat Cell Biol* 2006;8:384–90.

90   Danner S, Kajahn J, Geismann C *et al.* Derivation of oocyte-like cells from a clonal pancreatic stem cell line. *Mol Hum Reprod* 2007;13:11–20.

91   Feng LX, Chen Y, Dettin L *et al.* Generation and in vitro differentiation of a spermatogonial cell line. *Science* 2002;297:392–5.

92   Nayernia K, Nolte J, Michelmann HW *et al.* In vitro-differentiated embryonic stem cells give rise to male gametes that can generate offspring mice. *Dev Cell* 2006;11:125–32.

93   Roulet V, Denis H, Staub C *et al.* Human testis in organotypic culture: application for basic or clinical research. *Hum Reprod* 2006;21:1564–75.